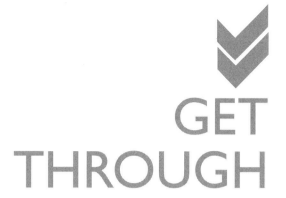

GET THROUGH

Primary FRCA:
MTFs

T0172402

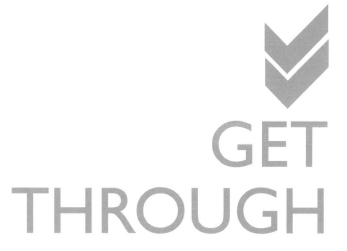

GET
THROUGH

Primary FRCA:
MTFs

James Day MBChB (Hons) FRCA
Specialty Registrar Anaesthetics, Oxford Deanery, Oxford, UK

Amy Thomson MBChB, FRCA (Primary), MRCP (Parts 1 & 2)
Specialty Registrar, Severn Deanery, UK

Tamsin McAllister MBChB (Hons) BMedSc
Specialty Registrar Anaesthetics, Oxford Deanery, UK

Nawal Bahal MBBS (Lond) BSc (Hons) FRCA
Consultant Anaesthetist
The Royal London Hospital, London, UK

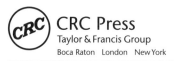

CRC Press
Taylor & Francis Group
Boca Raton   London   New York

CRC Press is an imprint of the
Taylor & Francis Group, an **informa** business

CRC Press
Taylor & Francis Group
6000 Broken Sound Parkway NW, Suite 300
Boca Raton, FL 33487-2742

© 2014 by James Day, Amy Thomson, and Tamsin McAllister
CRC Press is an imprint of Taylor & Francis Group, an Informa business

No claim to original U.S. Government works

Printed on acid-free paper
Version Date: 20140411

International Standard Book Number-13: 978-1-4441-8178-4 (Paperback)

Visit the Taylor & Francis Web site at
http://www.taylorandfrancis.com

and the CRC Press Web site at
http://www.crcpress.com

CONTENTS

ACKNOWLEDGMENTS

The authors would like to thank the following individuals for their support over the years.

JD: For Fiona, Isabella and Sophie
TM: For Rob, my Mum and Dad, Kiera, Marcus and my Gran
AT: For Donald and Fiona
NB: For Rachel

In addition, we are grateful for the support of the following doctors. The successes we have enjoyed have been built on their input and hard work over the years, for which we remain indebted: Alastair Ankers, Marc Davison, Maria Okoisor, Andrew Papanikitas, Rob Paul, Elize Richards, Stephen Snyders and Steven Webster-Edge.

Finally, we would like to thank our editors at Taylor & Francis/CRC Press. In particular, Stephen Clausard, who has been instrumental throughout the production of the book. We are all very grateful for the hard work, dedication and patience you have demonstrated.

INTRODUCTION

After the successes of *Get Through Final FRCA: MCQs* and the examdoctor.co.uk website, it was always my plan to move on to create an MCQ book for the Primary FRCA. In many ways this is an exam like no other. It is notoriously difficult for a start. Where other subspecialties in medicine have been accused of 'lowering the bar', even the sharpest of hawks in anaesthesia will concede that the Primary FRCA remains a very difficult exam.

Preparation must occur whilst learning and applying new skills, balancing the need for practical experience and study. It is also more than anaesthesia. Most anaesthetists will complete their training and their career having never used ether, or relied on their knowledge of precisely how a LASER is generated. These questions can seem cruel when balancing working over weekends and nights, exam preparation and (hopefully) a personal life.

Writing as someone who has recently completed training, I can tell you that it is all worth it. The FRCA takes a lot out of you over the first few years of training but the rewards are vast, not least the confidence of being able to apply your knowledge to all manner of tasks. The FRCA is your framework for the rest of your career.

James Day and I were editors for examdoctor, and it took us no time to select the authors we wanted to work with for this book. James Day, Amy Thomson and Tamsin McAllister have been excellent authors and have taken great care to cover the entire FRCA syllabus. In addition, they have stuck with the Hodder formula of including references for further reading with each question for those who wish to use the question as a platform for further reading. They should take a lot of pride in having produced an excellent body of work.

In addition to the five papers, we have included a special section that summarizes many of the formulae, units and normal values required in your learning. Although the list is by no means exhaustive, we believe that this chapter will be useful for both the written component and the Structured Oral Examinations (SOEs).

I have enjoyed editing this book and have learned much that I confess I did not know. I hope you find it a valuable resource.

Good luck for your forthcoming exam and beyond.

Nawal Bahal, MBBS (Lond) BSc (Hons) FRCA
Consultant Anaesthetist
The Royal London Hospital

FORMULAE FOR THE FRCA

Included in the following are a number of units, formulae and normal values pertinent to both parts of the FRCA examination. Whilst not exhaustive, we hope that the following section will be helpful in preparation for the MCQ, SAQ and SOE components.

PHYSICS

SI Units

Base
Amount of substance (*mole*, mol)
Electrical current (*ampere*, A)
Length (*metre*, m)
Luminous intensity (*candela*, cd)
Mass (*kilogram*, kg)
Thermodynamic temperature (*kelvin*, K)
Time (*second*, s)

Derived (derivation from SI base units included)
Angle (no dimension, *radian*, rad)
Electrical capacitance ($kg^{-1} \cdot m^{-2} \cdot s^4 \cdot A^2$, *farad*, F)
Electrical charge ($A \cdot s$, *coulomb*, C)
Electrical resistance ($kg \cdot m^2 \cdot s^{-3} \cdot A^{-2}$, *ohm*, Ω)
Force ($kg \cdot m \cdot s^{-2}$, *newton*, N)
Frequency (s^{-1}, *hertz*, Hz)
Magnetic field strength ($kg \cdot s^{-2} \cdot A^{-1}$, *tesla*, T)
Magnetic flux ($kg \cdot m^2 \cdot s^{-2} \cdot A^{-1}$, *weber*, Wb)
Potential difference ($kg \cdot m^2 \cdot s^{-3} \cdot A^{-1}$, *volt*, V)
Power ($kg \cdot m^2 \cdot s^{-3}$, *watt*, W)
Pressure ($kg \cdot m^{-1} \cdot s^{-2}$, *pascal*, Pa)
Work, energy and heat ($kg \cdot m^2 \cdot s^{-2}$, *joule*, J)

Pressure

1 atmosphere (atm) = 101.3 kPa
= 760 mmHg
= 760 torr
= 14.7 lb·square inch^{-1}
= 1033 cmH$_2$O
= 1.013 bar

Capacitance

C = Q/V
C = capacitance (*farad*), V = potential difference (*volt*), Q = charge (*coulomb*)

Ohm's law

R = V/I
R = resistance (*ohm*), V = potential difference, I = current (*ampere*)

Power in watts

P = IV
P = power (*watt*), I = current, V = potential difference

Fick principle

Cardiac output = Oxygen consumption/Arterial – Mixed venous oxygen
concentration

Laplace's law

P = T/R for a cylinder
P = 2T/R for a sphere
P = transmural pressure, T = wall tension (*newton*), R = radius

Hagen–Poiseuille law

Q = ΔPr^4/8ηL
Q = laminar flow through a tube, ΔP = pressure gradient across the length of the tube,
r = radius of the tube, η = viscosity of the fluid (Pa·s^{-1}), L = length of the tube

PHYSIOLOGY

Anion gap

([Na$^+$] + [K$^+$]) – ([HCO$_3^-$] + [Cl$^-$])
Normal values
5–12 mmol·L^{-1}

Osmolality

2(Na$^+$ + K$^+$) + Urea + Glucose
Note that this calculation is an approximation. Normal values: 285–295 mOsm·kg^{-1}

Starling equation

$Q = \kappa\,([P_c - P_i] - \sigma[\pi_c - \pi_i])$

Q = flow, κ = filtration coefficient, σ = reflection coefficient, P_c = capillary hydrostatic pressure, π_c = interstitial fluid colloid osmotic pressure, P_i = interstitial fluid hydrostatic pressure, π_i = capillary colloid osmotic pressure

Nernst equation

$E = RT/zF$

E = equilibrium potential of the ion (*volts*), R = universal gas constant ($8.3144621\ \mathrm{J \cdot K^{-1} \cdot mol^{-1}}$), T = absolute temperature (*kelvin*), z = valency of the ion, F = Faraday's constant ($9.64853399 \times 10^4\ \mathrm{C \cdot mol^{-1}}$)

Cerebral perfusion pressure (CPP)

$CPP = MAP - (ICP + CVP)$

Body mass index (BMI)

$BMI = Weight/Height^2$
Weight in kilograms, height in metres

WHO ranges for BMI

<15 = Very severely underweight
15–16 = Severely underweight
16–18.5 = Underweight
18.5–25 = Normal (healthy weight)
25–30 = Overweight
30–35 = Obese Class I (moderately obese)
35–40 = Obese Class II (severely obese)
>40 = Obese Class III (very severely obese)

Haemodynamics

Cardiac output (CO)

$CO = SV \times HR$
Normal adult values: 4.5–8 $\mathrm{L \cdot min^{-1}}$

Cardiac index (CI)

$CI = CO/Body\ surface\ area\ (BSA)$
Normal adult values: 3–3.5 $\mathrm{L \cdot min^{-1} \cdot m^{-2}}$

Stroke volume (SV)

SV = End diastolic (EDV) – End systolic volume (ESV)
Normal adult values: 70–120 ml

Stroke volume index (SI)

SV/BSA
Normal adult values: 30–50 $\mathrm{ml \cdot m^{-2}}$

Systemic vascular resistance (SVR)

$SVR = 80 \times (MAP - CVP)/CO$

Normal adult values: 900–1400 dyn·s^{-1}·cm^{-5}

Systemic vascular resistance index (SVRI)

$SVRI = 80 \times (MAP - CVP)/CI$

Normal adult values: 1800–2500 dyn·s^{-1}·cm^{-5}

Pulmonary vascular resistance (PVR)

$PVR = 80 \times (MPAP - LAP)/CO$

Normal adult values: 100–250 dyn·s^{-1}·cm^{-5}

Ejection fraction (EF)

$EF = (SV/EDV) \times 100$

Normal adult values: >60%

Normal adult values for cardiovascular pressures (mmHg)

CVP: 0–8

Right atrium: 1–4

Right ventricle: 25/4

Pulmonary artery: 25/12

Pulmonary capillary wedge pressure (PCWP): 6–12

Left atrium: 2–10

Left ventricle: 120/10

Aorta: 120/70

Renal

Creatinine clearance

$CCr = U_{Creat}V/P_{Creat}$

CCr = urinary creatinine clearance, V = urine flow, P_{Creat} = plasma creatinine concentration

Renal plasma flow (RPF)

$RPF = U_{PAH}V/P_{PAH}$

U_{PAH} = urinary concentration of PAH (para-aminohippuric acid), V = urine flow (ml·min^{-1}), P_{PAH} = plasma concentration of PAH

Respiratory

Shunt equation

$Q_S/Q_T = (CcO_2 - CaO_2)/(CcO_2 - CvO_2)$

Q_S = shunt flow, Q_T = total flow, CcO_2 = pulmonary capillary oxygen content, CaO_2 = arterial oxygen content, CvO_2 = mixed venous oxygen content

Lung volumes and capacities
(See the diagram in Chapter 6 [Paper 3], Answer 36)
FRC = RV + ERV
VC = TV + IRV + ERV
RV = FRC – ERV
TLC = FRC + TV + IRV or = VC+ RV

Oxygen content
$CaO_2 = (1.34 \times Hb \times SaO_2)/100 + 0.023 \times PaO_2$
0.023 is the solubility coefficient of O_2 in blood at 37°C giving the O_2 carried in
blood in ml·dL^{-1}·kPa^{-1}. 1.34 is the Hüfner constant giving the oxygen content of
1 g of fully saturated haemoglobin.

Oxygen saturation
O_2 content of Hb × 100/O_2 capacity of Hb

Oxygen flux (delivery)
Cardiac output × Arterial oxygen content

Physiological dead space (Bohr's method)
$V_D/V_T = (P_AO_2 – P_EO_2)/P_ACO_2$
V_D = dead space, V_T = tidal volume, P_AO_2 = alveolar oxygen tension, P_EO_2 =
expired oxygen tension, P_ACO_2 = alveolar CO_2 tension

Alveolar gas equation
$P_AO_2 = FiO_2 (P_B – P_AH_2O) – P_ACO_2/RQ$
P_AO_2 = alveolar oxygen tension, P_B = barometric pressure, P_AH_2O = SVP of water
at body temperature and the measured atmospheric pressure, RQ = respiratory
quotient (CO_2 eliminated/O_2 consumed)

PHARMACOLOGY

Rate of diffusion (Fick's law)
$Q – K_pAC/T$
Q = diffusion flux (mol·m^{-2}·s^{-1}), K_p = membrane permeability, C = concentration
difference, A = area of membrane, T = membrane thickness

Therapeutic index
Median lethal dose/Median effective dose

Henderson-Hasselbalch equation
Derived from the acid dissociation constant.

$K_a = [H^+][A^-]/[HA]$
$\log_{10} K_a = \log_{10} ([H^+][A^-]/[HA])$
$\log_{10} K_a = \log_{10} [H^+] + \log_{10} ([A^-]/[HA])$

$-pK_a = -pH + \log_{10} ([A^-]/[HA])$
$\therefore pH = pK_a + \log_{10} ([A^-]/[HA])$
K_a = dissociation constant

PAPER I
QUESTIONS

1. Ketamine:
   A. Has a pKa of 7.5
   B. Has two geometric stereoisomers
   C. Is more lipid soluble than thiopentone
   D. Has local anaesthetic properties
   E. Effects are mediated by central agonism at the N-methyl-D-aspartate (NMDA) receptor

2. When compared with atracurium, cisatracurium:
   A. Is more potent
   B. Has fewer autonomic side effects
   C. Causes less histamine release
   D. Produces more laudanosine
   E. Has a slower onset time

3. Lignocaine:
   A. Prolongs the duration of the cardiac action potential
   B. Acts on the intracellular portion of the ligand-gated sodium channel
   C. Possesses a COO group
   D. Causes methaemoglobinaemia in infants
   E. Is 95% protein-bound

4. The metabolism of the following drugs is influenced by hepatic blood flow:
   A. Propranolol
   B. Phenytoin
   C. Warfarin
   D. Tricyclic antidepressants
   E. Morphine

5. There is increased risk of bleeding when:
   A. Aspirin is administered with ibuprofen
   B. Aspirin is administered with clopidogrel
   C. Any patient is taking clopidogrel
   D. An abciximab infusion has been stopped 72 hours ago
   E. The bleeding time is 4 minutes

6. Insulin:
A. Is produced commercially using recombinant DNA technology
B. Is combined with protamine to delay subcutaneous absorption
C. Is only metabolized in the liver
D. Is removed by dialysis
E. Has little protein binding

7. Aspirin:
A. Has a pKa of 5.3
B. Is 90% protein-bound
C. Is a prodrug
D. Causes metabolic alkalosis in overdose
E. Increases cellular oxygen consumption

8. The following agents inhibit cyclo-oxygenase enzymes:
A. Phenylbutazone
B. Papaveretum
C. Tenoxicam
D. Pentazocine
E. Etoricoxib

9. The following pairings of antibiotics and effect sites are correct:
A. Erythromycin and 30S ribosome subunit
B. Aminoglycosides and 30S ribosome unit
C. Cephalosporins and peptidoglycan cell wall
D. Quinolones and DNA-gyrase
E. Rifampicin and elongation factor

10. The following drugs are removed by haemodialysis:
A. Sodium nitroprusside
B. Penicillin
C. Morphine
D. Amitriptyline
E. Temazepam

11. Midazolam:
A. Is metabolized to an inactive metabolite
B. Is removed by renal replacement therapy
C. Has a shorter half-life than lorazepam
D. Is potentiated when given with clarithromycin
E. Binds at a site between the α and γ subunits of the $GABA_A$ receptor

12. Regarding paracetamol:
A. It has a maximum safe dosage of 4 g in 24 hours for those over 16 years of age
B. Overdose is the most common cause of acute liver failure worldwide
C. It is a cyclo-oxygenase inhibitor
D. It has good bioavailability as a rectal suppository
E. It is synthesized from phenol

13. Side effects of amiodarone include:
A. Bradycardia
B. Hypothyroidism
C. Jaundice
D. Nephrotoxicity
E. Prolonged QT interval

14. Cimetidine:
A. Is an imidazole derivative
B. Induces hepatic cytochrome P450
C. Is a competitive antagonist at H_2 receptors
D. 90% is excreted in urine unchanged
E. Increases metabolism of phenytoin

15. Drugs that inhibit monoamine oxidase (MAO) include:
A. Ephedrine
B. Linezolid
C. Moclobemide
D. Hydralazine
E. Isoniazid

16. Remifentanil:
A. Has activity at μ- and κ-opioid receptors
B. Has a fixed context-sensitive half-time of 3–5 minutes
C. Reaches peak effect after 5–10 minutes
D. Is less potent than fentanyl
E. Should be avoided in renal impairment due to active metabolites

17. Passive diffusion is increased by:
A. High molecular weight
B. Low lipid solubility
C. Ionization
D. Plasma protein binding
E. Large concentration gradient

18. Smoking cessation:
A. The night before surgery does not reduce carbon monoxide levels
B. After 6 weeks reduces postoperative pulmonary complication rate to that of non-smokers
C. For 12 hours increases physical work capacity by 10–20%
D. Reduces upper airway irritability after 12 hours
E. Within 2 months of surgery shows no positive effects

19. The following β-blockers are selective for the $β_1$-receptor:
A. Propranolol
B. Metoprolol
C. Acebutalol
D. Atenolol
E. Sotalol

20. The following diuretics do not cause hypokalaemia:
A. Amiloride
B. Spironolactone
C. Bumetanide
D. Metolazone
E. Bendroflumethiazide

21. The following are derived SI units:
A. Volt
B. Farad
C. Hertz
D. Kilogram
E. Mole

22. The following statements about humidity are correct:
A. Absolute humidity, measured in $mg \cdot m^{-2}$, is the amount of water vapour present in a given volume of gas
B. Relative humidity, measured in percent (%), is the ratio of the amount of water vapour present in a gas, compared with the mass of water required to saturate the gas at the same temperature
C. At 37°C and 100% relative humidity, the absolute humidity of air is 44 $g \cdot m^{-3}$
D. The temperature at which the relative humidity of a gas exceeds 100% is the dew point
E. At 50% relative humidity, air cannot contain 44 $g \cdot m^{-3}$ of water vapour until it reaches 50°C

23. Viscosity:
A. Is the property of a fluid that resists flow
B. Of a fluid can be described by its coefficient of viscosity, which is determined by shear rate and damping
C. Of a gas increases with increasing temperature
D. Of a Newtonian fluid is constant, regardless of its shear rate
E. Will make laminar flow more likely for a gas, if increased

24. The following statements are correct:
A. The Doppler effect is the phenomenon by which the frequency of transmitted sound is altered as it is reflected from an object moving away from the receiver
B. The oesophageal Doppler calculates the volume of blood in the descending aorta
C. The velocity of sound in blood is 1570 $m \cdot s^{-1}$
D. 90% of cardiac output passes through the descending aorta
E. The Doppler equation can be used to calculate the pressure gradient across the aortic valve

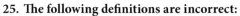

25. The following definitions are incorrect:
A. Power (joules) is work done per unit time
B. Work (joules) is force exerted multiplied by the distance travelled in the direction of the force
C. Force (newtons) is equal to mass multiplied by velocity
D. Cardiac work is equal to pressure multiplied by volume
E. One newton is the force that will increase the velocity of one kilogram by one metre per second every second ($kg \cdot m \cdot s^{-2}$)

26. Pulse oximetry:
A. Uses two light-emitting diodes that transmit light at 660 and 810 nm
B. Is based on the Stewart–Hamilton law
C. Has limited accuracy with tricuspid regurgitation
D. Is not affected by jaundice
E. Is not accurate in neonates due to presence of foetal haemoglobin

27. The following statements are correct:
A. As fluid flowing along a tube enters a constriction, the velocity of fluid flow will increase
B. Bernoulli's equation for incompressible flow relates pressure, velocity and viscosity of a fluid
C. The second law of thermodynamics states that energy in a system cannot be created or destroyed but instead must change from one form to another
D. The entrainment ratio is calculated as driving flow/entrained flow
E. The Venturi effect describes the effect by which the introduction of a constriction to fluid flow in a tube will cause the pressure of the fluid to fall

28. In a parallel circuit:
A. The same current flows around the whole circuit
B. The circuit's resistance is calculated by adding the individual resistances together
C. The total capacitance is calculated by adding the individual capacitors together
D. Electrons flow from positive to negative
E. The current flowing can be calculated as voltage multiplied by resistance

29. The Manley MP3 ventilator:
A. Has two unidirectional valves
B. Its oxygen flush can safely be used
C. Has a pressure monitoring alarm on the expiratory limb
D. Functions as a Mapleson B during spontaneous ventilation
E. Is a minute volume divider

30. The following devices function using the Venturi effect:
A. Variable performance oxygen masks
B. Nebulizers
C. Gas cylinders
D. Vacuum cleaners
E. Jet ventilators

31. **Which of the following electrical components are found in a defibrillator?**
    A. Capacitor
    B. Transformer
    C. Resistor
    D. Inductor
    E. Diode

32. **The following statements are correct concerning the measurement of temperature:**
    A. The Fahrenheit scale is based on the properties of water
    B. The Celsius scale was developed using the mercury thermometer
    C. A degree on the Kelvin scale has the same magnitude as a degree on the Celsius scale
    D. The kelvin is the SI unit of temperature
    E. The kelvin is defined as equal to 1/273.16 of the absolute temperature of the triple point of water

33. **The following are correct regarding the safety features of gas cylinders:**
    A. They are made from manganese steel
    B. Oxygen cylinders are black with a white shoulder
    C. A pin index system is used to prevent accidental connection of a cylinder to the wrong yoke on the anaesthetic machine
    D. In a fire, a cylinder will inevitably explode
    E. The type of gas is written on the cylinder

34. **The following statements are correct regarding electricity supply in the United Kingdom:**
    A. Direct current has a frequency of 10 Hz
    B. The maximum voltage of mains electricity is 240 V
    C. The frequency of mains supply has been chosen to minimize the risk of electric shock
    D. A standard electrical supply wire contains three conductors
    E. Resistive power loss is affected by the transmission current

35. **Regarding electrical safety:**
    A. Class I equipment relies on fuses in the live and neutral wire
    B. Class II equipment still needs three wires in the electrical cable
    C. Class III equipment has no risk of electric shock associated with mains electricity
    D. In CF equipment, C stands for 'cardiac' and F for 'floating'
    E. CF equipment has a maximum permissible leakage current of 50 µA

36. **A lignocaine spray that delivers 10 mg of the drug in each 0.1 ml spray is of the following concentration:**
    A. 1%
    B. 0.1%
    C. 10%
    D. 100%
    E. 5%

37. The following are or contain a semi-conductor:
A. Electrical fuse
B. Silicon
C. Thermistor
D. Diode
E. Transformer

38. Regarding biological electrical signals:
A. The electromyogram (EMG) potential from a motor neurone of the medial rectus muscle is greater than from the rectus femoris muscle
B. Electrocardiogram (ECG) potential is around 90 mV
C. Electroencephalogram (EEG) potential is around 1–2 mV
D. The potential measured from the electromyogram has a much shorter duration than those from the electrocardiogram
E. The range of potentials measured from an electromyogram may differ by 1000-fold in magnitude

39. Capacitance:
A. Is measured in coulombs
B. Is greater as the distance between the two conducting plates in a capacitor is increased
C. Is the result of Charge (Q) × Potential difference (V)
D. Energy in a capacitor = ½ Capacitance (C) × Potential difference (V)
E. Is the ability of a structure to store electrical charge

40. When using the thermodilution technique of cardiac output monitoring:
A. Cold saline is injected via the distal port of the pulmonary artery catheter
B. Change in temperature is detected by a thermocouple in the catheter tip
C. The thermodilution principle utilizes the Stewart–Hamilton equation
D. A second peak, known as a recirculation hump, is seen on the temperature vs time graph
E. Accuracy is affected by blood temperature variations

41. Potassium:
A. Is 85% intracellular
B. Is predominantly stored in skeletal muscle
C. Is the second most abundant intracellular cation
D. Is predominantly reabsorbed in the proximal convoluted tubule
E. From dietary intake is absorbed in the large intestine

42. The human kidney:
A. Contains more than 2 million nephrons
B. Produces 180 L·day^{-1} of glomerular filtrate
C. Receives 30% of cardiac output at rest
D. Has a filtration fraction of 20%
E. Receives 200 ml·100 g^{-1}·min^{-1} blood flow

43. Sympathetic stimulation of the heart:
A. Increases intracellular cyclic AMP
B. Decreases reuptake of calcium into sarcoplasmic reticulum
C. Increases myosin cross-bridge formation
D. Increases potassium permeability at the sino-atrial node
E. Increases activation of L-type calcium channels in ventricular myocytes

44. Pulmonary vascular resistance:
A. Is approximately 10% of the systemic vascular resistance
B. Is determined by muscular arterioles
C. Increases as pulmonary arterial pressure increases
D. Is decreased at low lung volumes in extra-alveolar vessels
E. Decreases with exercise

45. The following physiological changes occur during a Valsalva manoeuvre:
A. An initial fall in mean arterial pressure
B. Increased intra-abdominal pressure resulting in reduced venous return to the heart
C. Increased stimulation of baroreceptors resulting in reflex tachycardia
D. Reduced intrathoracic pressure, which immediately increases blood pressure
E. On releasing Valsalva, blood pressure overshoots due to reflex bradycardia

46. Regarding types of nerve fibres:
A. Aβ fibres transmit touch and temperature sensation
B. C fibres transmit pain sensation
C. Aγ fibres are found in the autonomic nervous system
D. B fibres are postganglionic autonomic fibres
E. Aα fibres are somatic motor neurones

47. For glucose metabolism:
A. Pyruvate generation requires oxygen
B. The glycolytic pathway generates six molecules of adenosine triphosphate (ATP)
C. The glycolytic pathway uses two molecules of ATP
D. The citric acid cycle takes place in cell cytoplasm
E. Under aerobic conditions, 1 mole of glucose can generate 32 moles of ATP

48. The following will increase cerebral blood flow:
A. Mean arterial pressure increase from 90 to 140 mmHg
B. Decrease in PaO_2 to 8 kPa
C. Increase in $PaCO_2$ to 6 kPa
D. Increase in the cerebral metabolic requirement for oxygen
E. Increase in cerebral metabolic glucose consumption

49. Hydrochloric acid secretion in the stomach:
   A. Is from the chief cells
   B. Is stimulated by histamine
   C. Helps the absorption of calcium
   D. Is reduced by glycopyrrolate
   E. Is increased by somatostatin

50. Liver blood supply:
   A. Is approximately 25% of total resting cardiac output
   B. Comes from the hepatic portal vein and the hepatic vein
   C. Is approximately 1.5 L·min⁻¹ in a 70 kg adult
   D. Through the parenchyma has the bile duct at the centre of the hepatic lobule
   E. Has partially passed through the spleen

51. Regarding the sympathetic nervous system:
   A. The sympathetic trunk runs bilaterally from the first thoracic vertebra to the second lumbar vertebra
   B. The stellate ganglion is the name given to the fusion of the inferior cervical ganglion with the first thoracic ganglion
   C. Cell bodies of the preganglionic neurones lie within the lateral horn of the spinal cord
   D. All of the preganglionic neurones synapse within the sympathetic trunk
   E. The preganglionic neurones synapse in the sympathetic trunk via the grey ramus communicans

52. The bronchopulmonary segment of the lung:
   A. Total of 12 in each lung
   B. Are supplied by tertiary bronchi
   C. Possesses dual arterial supply
   D. Possesses venous drainage that runs through the centre of the segment
   E. Are separated by a layer of connective tissue and can be surgically resected

53. In the eye:
   A. The posterior chamber is anterior to the iris
   B. The anterior chamber is posterior to the cornea
   C. The anterior and posterior chambers are filled with vitreous humour
   D. The ciliary muscle is innervated by parasympathetic fibres via the oculomotor nerve
   E. Contraction of the ciliary muscle tightens the suspensory ligaments and flattens the lens increasing the refractive power

54. The following statements about the blood supply of the brain are correct:
   A. It is supplied by four arteries
   B. The middle cerebral artery is part of the posterior circulation
   C. The circle of Willis contains two anterior communicating arteries and one posterior communicating artery
   D. The basilar artery is formed by the fusion of the left and right vertebral arteries
   E. The middle cerebral artery supplies the lateral surface and temporal pole of the brain

55. Surfactant:

A. Is produced by type 1 alveolar cells
B. Increases pulmonary compliance
C. Increases alveolar surface tension
D. Is predominantly composed of carbohydrate molecules
E. Has a greater stabilizing effect on smaller alveoli

56. Maintenance of acid–base balance by the kidney occurs by:

A. Hydrogen ion secretion, primarily in the distal convoluted tubule
B. Reabsorption of bicarbonate in the proximal convoluted tubule
C. Excretion of hydrogen ions as ammonia
D. Hydrogen ion secretion in combination with cations in the tubular fluid
E. Active secretion of hydrogen ions in the distal convoluted tubule

57. For aerobic metabolism of glucose:

A. The Pasteur point is 0.4 kPa
B. The main form of energy produced by glucose metabolism is ATP
C. A net total of 38 ATP molecules are produced by aerobic metabolism of one glucose molecule
D. The Krebs cycle takes place on the outer mitochondrial membrane
E. The entry point for acetyl CoA into the Krebs cycle is in combination with oxaloacetate to form citric acid

58. Regarding muscarinic receptors:

A. They are pentameric ion channels
B. They are G-protein-coupled receptors
C. The M1 subtypes increase potassium conductance in the sino-atrial node
D. The M2 subtypes are found in atrial tissue
E. Stimulation of the M1 receptor increases gastric acid secretion

59. The following are true of the intrinsic pathway of the classical coagulation cascade:

A. Factor 10 is inactivated under the influence of tissue factor and activated factor 7
B. The activation of factor 9 is calcium-dependent
C. Factor 11 is activated under the influence of fibrinogen
D. Factor 5 activates factor 10
E. Activated factor 11 activates factor 9

60. The following hormones act at G-protein-coupled receptors:

A. Oxytocin
B. Glucagon
C. Insulin
D. Thyroxine
E. Adrenaline

PAPER 1
ANSWERS

1A: True
1B: False
1C: True
1D: True
1E: False

Ketamine is a phencyclidine derivative, which has many indications for use. It is used for the induction of general anaesthesia, as an analgesic agent, to provide analgesia and sedation for short procedures, as an adjunct in epidural anaesthesia and in the management of severe asthma.

Ketamine typically causes dissociative anaesthesia and has a number of benefits, including analgesic properties, maintenance of airway tone and spontaneous ventilation with cardiovascular stability. The major drawback of ketamine as an anaesthetic agent is its association with emergence reactions, delirium, hallucinations and vivid dreams.

The main mechanism of action of ketamine is interaction with the phencyclidine binding site at the N-methyl-D-aspartate (NMDA) receptor, resulting in non-competitive antagonism of L-glutamate (a major excitatory neurotransmitter in the central nervous system). Ketamine also has local anaesthetic properties in high doses (sodium channel blockade) along with interaction at opioid, monoaminergic, muscarinic and nicotinic receptors.

Ketamine has a chiral centre with two optical stereoisomers: R- and S-ketamine. The pKa of ketamine is 7.5. Ketamine is highly lipid soluble (up to 10 times more soluble than thiopentone) and penetrates the blood–brain barrier rapidly. S-ketamine is the more potent enantiomer, with fewer side effects, shorter recovery time and greater affinity for the NMDA receptor.

Further reading

Pai A, Heining M. Ketamine. *Contin Educ Anaesth Crit Care Pain*. 2003; 7(2): 59–63.

Smith S, Scarth E, Sasada M. *Drugs in Anaesthesia and Intensive Care*. 4th ed. Oxford: Oxford University Press; 2011.

2A: True
2B: True
2C: True
2D: False
2E: True

Atracurium possesses four chiral molecules. Ten stereoisomers may exist, one of which is cisatracurium. Cisatracurium is more potent than atracurium (four times more potent), produces fewer autonomic side effects and releases less histamine. As cisatracurium is more potent, a lower dose of the drug is required, resulting in less laudanosine production. The onset of action of cisatracurium is slow; however, the dose can be increased to speed the rate of onset (Bowman's principle). Like atracurium, cisatracurium is metabolized by Hoffman elimination and ester hydrolysis and has no active metabolites.

Further reading

Appiah-Ankam J, Hunter JH. Pharmacology of neuromuscular blocking drugs. *Contin Educ Anaesth Crit Care Pain.* 2004; 4(1): 2–7.

3A: False
3B: False
3C: False
3D: False
3E: False

Lignocaine is an amide local anaesthetic agent, composed of a lipophilic aromatic group and a hydrophilic amine group joined by an amide link (NH-CO). Local anaesthetic agents act on the intracellular portion of the voltage-gated sodium channel where a blockade prevents the spread of action potentials in excitable cells. Lignocaine has both local anaesthetic and anti-arrhythmic properties. Lignocaine is a class 1b anti-arrhythmic agent, blocking the voltage-gated sodium channel in the cardiac cell. Class 1b agents shorten the repolarization phase of the action potential, reducing re-entry phenomena, and are used for their membrane stabilizing effects in the management of ventricular arrhythmias.

Lignocaine has a pKa of 7.9, so is largely unionized at physiological pH with a rapid onset time. Lignocaine is 70% protein-bound. O-toludine, a metabolite of the amide local anaesthetic agent prilocaine, causes methaemoglobinaemia in infants; however, lignocaine is not known to have this effect.

Further reading

Whiteside, JB, Wildsmith JAW. *Preparing for the Primary FRCA: Local Anaesthetics.* Bulletin 2, The Royal College of Anaesthetists; 2000. p. 64–67.

4A: True
4B: False
4C: False
4D: True
4E: True

Hepatic metabolism of drugs is influenced by the saturability (i.e. capacity) of the metabolizing enzymes and the delivery of the drug to the hepatocyte (hepatic blood flow). The rate of hepatic metabolism is referred to as the hepatic extraction ratio (ER). Metabolizing enzymes with a high Michaelis constant (the concentration of substrate at which the enzyme is working at 50% maximum rate) have a high capacity for metabolizing the drug, thus the hepatic ER will be influenced by the delivery of the drug to the liver in the hepatic blood flow. The metabolism of these drugs is therefore 'flow dependent'. Flow-dependent drug metabolism (with high hepatic ER) is seen with propranolol, propofol, tricyclic antidepressants, opioids and lignocaine.

Metabolizing enzymes with a low Michaelis constant have a low capacity for drug metabolism, resulting in a low hepatic ER. Any increase in the free unbound fraction of the drug reaching the hepatocyte will readily saturate the enzyme system. This has clinical implications if the drug is highly protein-bound (where a small change in protein binding results in a largely proportional increase in free drug) and if the drug has a low therapeutic window. The metabolism of these drugs is therefore 'capacity limited'. Capacity-limited drug metabolism is seen with phenytoin, warfarin, barbiturates, NSAIDs and benzodiazepines.

Further reading

Remmer H. The role of the liver in drug metabolism. *Am J Med.* 1970; 49(5): 617–629.

5A: False
5B: True
5C: False
5D: False
5E: False

When concurrent administration of non-steroidal anti-inflammatory drugs (NSAIDs) occurs, there is competition with aspirin for the active binding site, which reduces aspirin bioavailability leading to aspirin resistance. Dual therapy of clopidogrel and aspirin leads to an increased risk of bleeding. This risk has been quoted as up to a 40% increase. In some patients, however, there is little effect when clopidogrel is taken. It is thought that up to 25% have a partial effect with 5–10% being resistant to its effect. This is likely to be due to a number of factors such as genetic differences in the P2Y12 receptor and activity in the P450 enzymes.

Abciximab (ReoPro™) is a GP IIb/IIIa receptor antagonist. The drug is given as a loading dose followed by an infusion. Its effects are active for up to 48 hours after termination of the infusion. The clinical effects of antiplatelets can be tested using point-of-care platelet function analyzers such as the thromboelastogram (TEG) and rotational thromboelastometry (ROTEM). The first test of platelet function was the bleeding time, developed in 1934. The test involves making an incision to produce a cut of a standard depth and width. A sphygmomanometer cuff is inflated to a pressure of 40 mmHg, and the time taken for bleeding to stop is noted. The normal times are quoted as between 2 and 10 minutes.

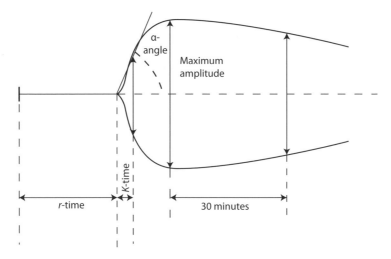

Thromboelastogram

The five parameters demonstrated are:

● *r*-time (reaction time) (15–30 min): Time from initiation of test until amplitude reaches 2 mm (initial fibrin formation)
● *K*-time (6–12 min): Time from *r*-time until amplitude reaches 20 mm – clot formation time
● α-angle (40–50°): Tangent of the curve as *K* is reached – speed at which clot forms
● MA (maximum amplitude) (50–60 mm): Greatest amplitude on the curve – 'maximal clot strength'
● LY30 (<7.5%): Based on area under curve 30 min after MA – measure of fibrinolysis

Further reading

Smart S, Aragola S, Hutton P. Antiplatelet agents and anaesthesia. *Contin Educ Anaesth Crit Care Pain*. 2007; 7(5): 157–161.

6A: **True**
6B: **True**
6C: **False**
6D: **False**
6E: **True**

The first genetically engineered synthetic insulin was produced in 1977, using *E. coli*. In 1982, Eli Lily commercially produced this biosynthetic insulin under the brand name Humulin. Untreated insulin has a rapid onset of action, exerting an effect within 1 hour and lasting for 4–5 hours. Combination with protamine or zinc extends the duration of action to 24 hours. Insulin is metabolized in the liver, muscle and kidney by glutathione insulin transhydrogenase. Insulin is not removed by dialysis. Insulin has little protein binding.

Further reading

Smith S, Scarth E, Sasada M. *Drugs in Anaesthesia and Intensive Care.* 4th ed. Oxford: Oxford University Press; 2011. p. 130–131.

7A: False
7B: True
7C: True
7D: False
7E: True

Aspirin is a salicylate, an aromatic ester of acetic acid, which is used for its antiplatelet, analgesic, anti-inflammatory and antipyretic effects. The drug is available in oral preparation only, at a dose range of 75–600 mg. The pKa of aspirin is 3.5. Aspirin acts by reducing prostaglandin and thromboxane production through inhibition of cyclo-oxygenase (COX) enzymes, with slight selectivity for the *COX-1* isoform. At the lower dose (75 mg), there is selective reduction in thromboxane production, causing selective antiplatelet effects. Systemic effects of aspirin include uncoupling of oxidative phosphorylation causing increased cellular oxygen consumption and increased carbon dioxide production. In overdose, an early respiratory alkalosis results from direct stimulation of the respiratory centre. This is followed by a longer-lasting metabolic acidosis due to the presence of endogenous acids in the blood rather than the salicylate itself.

Aspirin is well absorbed from the gastrointestinal tract, with an oral bioavailability of 70%. Aspirin undergoes rapid ester hydrolysis in the plasma to salicylic acid, which is the active compound and is highly protein-bound (90%). Salicylic acid is metabolized in the liver before the conjugated metabolite is excreted in the urine. Approximately 15% of salicylic acid is excreted unchanged.

Further reading

DeVile MPJ, Foex P. Antiplatelet drugs, coronary stents and non-cardiac surgery. *Contin Educ Anaesth Crit Care Pain.* 2010, 10(6). 187–191.

8A: True
8B: False
8C: True
8D: False
8E: True

Non-steroidal anti-inflammatory drugs (NSAIDs) are used in the treatment of mild to moderate pain. They inhibit the cyclo-oxygenase (COX) enzyme, reducing the formation of prostaglandins and thromboxane from arachidonic acid. This results in analgesia and anti-inflammatory effects (reduced production of PGE_2 and $PGF2_a$), alongside antiplatelet effects (reduced thromboxane production).

The cyclo-oxygenase enzymes exist as two main isoforms: *COX-1* and *COX-2*. There also exists a *COX 3* isoenzyme but this is a variant of *COX 1* and has minimal activity in humans. *COX-1* is the constitutive form that is responsible for the production of prostaglandins that form the gastric mucosa and control renal perfusion. *COX-2* is induced at times of tissue injury as part of the inflammatory response. Agents that are selective for the *COX-2* isoenzyme are rofecoxib, celecoxib, valdecoxib, parecoxib, eterocoxib and lumoricoxib. Meloxicam is preferential (rather than selective) for the *COX-2* enzyme. When they were initially produced, the *COX-2* inhibitors were favoured as they significantly reduce the incidence of gastrointestinal side effects when compared with non-selective COX inhibitors. However, the VIGOR study revealed an increased risk of coronary and cerebrovascular events with selective *COX-2* inhibitors, which has limited their use.

Papveretum and Pentazocine are opioid agents and Tenoxicam is a non-selective COX inhibitor of the oxicam family. Phenylbutazone is an NSAID licensed for use in gout and arthritis in 1949. It was withdrawn, as it is associated with aplastic anaemia and neutropenia.

Further reading

Bombardier C, Laine L, Reicin A, et al. Comparison of upper gastrointestinal toxicity of rofecoxib and naproxen in patients with rheumatoid arthritis. *NEJM.* 2010; 343(21): 1520–1528.

MHRA. Cardiovascular safety of *COX-2* inhibitors and non-selective NSAIDs. 2012. [Online] Available from: http://www.mhra.gov.uk.

9A: False
9B: True
9C: True
9D: True
9E: False

Erythromycin is a macrolide antibiotic (termed because they contain a macrocyclic lactone ring). Macrolides have a similar spectrum of activity as pencillins so are often used in patients with a penicillin allergy. They act by inhibiting protein synthesis through their binding to the P site of the 50S ribosomal subunit. Aminoglycosides such as gentamicin bind to the 30S ribosomal subunit, blocking protein synthesis. Cephalosporins, together with penicillins, act by inhibiting cell wall synthesis. They competitively inhibit transpeptidases that are involved in the cross linking of the peptidoglycan cell wall. Quinolones such as ciprofloxacin inhibit the α subunit of DNA-gyrase. This is a topoisomerase enzyme involved in the supercoiling of DNA. Rifampicin is a rifamycin antibiotic that prevents DNA transcription by binding to the β subunit of RNA polymerase. Fusidic acid acts by binding to elongation factor, halting protein translocation.

Further reading

Peck TE, Hill SA, Williams M. *Pharmacology for Anaesthesia and Intensive Care.* 3rd ed. Cambridge: Cambridge University Press; 2009.

10A: True
10B: True
10C: False
10D: False
10E: False

Sodium nitroprusside and penicillins are removed by haemodialysis. Morphine, amitriptyline and temazepam are not removed by haemodialysis. Other drugs that are removed by dialysis include: ethanol, methanol, aspirin, lithium, barbiturates, gentamicin, cephalosporins and ethylene glycol. Some drugs are not removed by dialysis. These include digoxin, tricyclic antidepressants, β-blockers, sulphonylureas and phenytoin.

Further reading

Sasada M, Smith S. *Drugs in Anaesthesia and Intensive Care.* 3rd ed. Oxford: Oxford University Press; 2007.

11A: False
11B: False
11C: True
11D: True
11E: True

Midazolam is a benzodiazepine. Benzodiazepines bind at a site lying between the α and γ subunits of the $GABA_A$ receptor. This causes the receptor to become more permeable to chloride ions, which causes hyperpolarization of the neurone. This leads to the observed effects of sedation, hypnosis, anxiolysis and anti-epileptic action. Barbiturates bind solely at the α subunit. Midazolam has a shorter half-life than lorazepam and is metabolized by the cytochrome P450 enzyme family to an active metabolite: hydroxyl-midazolam glucronide. This metabolite is renally excreted and is partially removed by renal replacement therapy. Midazolam is hardly cleared by renal replacement therapy at all. Co-administration of some antimicrobials, such as fluconazole or macrolides, inhibit the cytochrome P450 system, leading to increased effects of midazolam.

Further reading

Borthwick M. Pharmacology and pharmacokinetics of sedative agents. *JICS.* 2008; 9(3): 253–254.

12A: True
12B: False
12C: True
12D: False
12E: True

Paracetamol is an acetanilide derivative and is synthesized from phenol. It is an analgesic for mild to moderate pain and is used as an antipyretic too. The mechanism of action is poorly understood. It was thought that paracetamol had

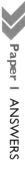
no effect on the cyclo-oxygenase (COX) enzyme but recent findings suggest that it is highly selective for COX₂? The adult dose is 4 g per day in divided doses. Paracetamol has good bioavailability as an oral preparation but has poor and variable bioavailability as a rectal preparation. It is the most common cause of acute liver failure in the United Kingdom but worldwide the most common cause is the hepatitis viruses.

Further reading

Oscier C, Milner Q. Peri-operative use of paracetamol. *Anaesthesia*. 2009; 64(1): 64–72.

13A: True
13B: True
13C: True
13D: False
13E: True
Amiodarone is a benzofuran derivative that can be used in the treatment of both ventricular and supraventricular tachyarrhythmias, as well as in the treatment of Wolff–Parkinson–White syndrome. It acts by blocking potassium channels, prolonging repolarization and thus increasing the duration of the action potential. It is a Vaughan–Williams class III anti-arrhythmic agent.

Amiodarone is given either by intravenous infusion or in tablet form. It is associated with a large number of side effects including:

- Raised serum transaminases and jaundice
- Hypo- and hyperthyroidism due to the prevention of peripheral conversion of T_3 to T_4
- Pneumonitis and fibrotic lung disease
- Photosensitivity and corneal micro deposits
- Tremor
- Bradycardia and prolongation of QT interval

Liver and thyroid function tests should be performed prior to commencement of treatment and every 6 months thereafter, and a chest X-ray should also be performed before starting treatment as a baseline.

Further reading

British National Formulary. London: BMJ Publishing Group and RPS Publishing; 2009. 58, 2.3.2, p. 84–85.

Peck TE, Hill SA, Williams M. *Pharmacology for Anaesthesia and Intensive Care*. 3rd ed. Cambridge: Cambridge University Press; 2008. Chapter 14, p. 238–239.

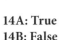

14A: True
14B: False
14C: True
14D: False
14E: False

Cimetidine is a competitive antagonist at parietal cell histamine (H_2) receptors, which are the main stimulus for gastric acid secretion. It has an imidazole structure and acts to inhibit gastric acid production, raising gastric pH and reducing volume of secretions.

It can be administered orally (60% bioavailability) or intravenously. On rapid intravenous bolus administration it can lead to bradycardia and hypotension.

It is metabolized in the liver by cytochrome P450 but 50% is excreted renally unchanged. In renal failure high plasma levels have been associated with hallucinations, confusion and seizures. Cimetidine is an inhibitor of hepatic cytochrome P450 and consequently increases the plasma levels of drugs metabolized by this route, including diazepam, phenytoin and warfarin.

It has anti-androgen effects, which can cause gynaecomastia, impotence and a drop in sperm count when used in male patients.

Further reading

Peck TE, Hill SA, Williams M. *Pharmacology for Anaesthesia and Intensive Care*. 3rd ed. Cambridge: Cambridge University Press; 2008. Chapter 19, p. 292–295.

15A: False
15B: True
15C: True
15D: True
15E: True

MAO is an enzyme involved in the metabolism of monoamines such as adrenaline, noradrenaline and dopamine and their precursors. It exists in two forms: MAO-A and MAO-B. MAO-A preferentially deaminates serotonin and catecholamines, whereas MAO-B preferentially deaminates tyramine and phenylethamine.

Drugs specifically designed to inhibit monoamine oxidase (MAO inhibitors, or MAOIs) are used in the treatment of depressive illnesses, obsessive-compulsive disorders, chronic pain syndromes and migraine. They include the non selective irreversible MAOIs phenelzine, isocarboxazid and tranylcypromine, and the selective reversible MAOI moclobemide. They prevent the metabolism of amine neurotransmitters, such as noradrenaline and serotonin; it is thought that depression is particularly related to reduced levels of serotonin in the central nervous systems of patients.

Patients taking MAOIs present a challenge to the anaesthetist as indirectly acting sympathomimetic agents such as ephedrine are reliant upon MAO for their metabolism, and their use can potentially result in exaggerated hypertension and life-threatening arrhythmias when used in the presence of MAOIs. Other drugs can also inhibit MAO and these should be used with particular caution in patients taking MAOIs.

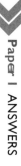
Drugs that inhibit MAO include:

- Hydralazine
- Isoniazid
- Linezolid
- Methylene blue

Further reading

Peck TE, Hill SA, Williams M. *Pharmacology for Anaesthesia and Intensive Care.* 3rd ed. Cambridge: Cambridge University Press; 2008. Chapter 17, p. 274–278.

Smith T, Pinnock C, Lin T (Ed). *Fundamentals of Anaesthesia.* 3rd ed. Cambridge: Cambridge University Press; 2009. Chapter 10, p. 640–641.

16A: False
16B: True
16C: False
16D: False
16E: False

Remifentanil is a synthetic phenylpiperidine derivative of fentanyl. It is a pure agonist at the μ-opioid receptor and is used for analgesia during general anaesthesia, labour, in intensive care and for procedures such as awake fibreoptic intubation.

It is ultra-short acting, being hydrolyzed rapidly by non-specific plasma and tissue esterases, so that its context-sensitive half-time is fixed at 3–5 minutes, regardless of duration of infusion. Consequently, it is not useful for postoperative analgesia as its effect wears off predictably within 5–10 minutes once the infusion is discontinued.

It reaches peak effect within 1–3 minutes and therefore can be rapidly titrated to effect.

Remifentanil is a potent respiratory depressant and also causes bradycardia and hypotension via centrally mediated vagal activity. It does not tend to cause nausea and vomiting and only has minimal hypnotic and sedative activity. It has an analgesic potency similar to fentanyl and is safe to use in renal and hepatic impairment as, although the metabolite, remifentanil acid, is a μ-opioid agonist, it has 4600-fold less activity and has not been shown to cause significant clinical effects, even though it may accumulate in renal failure.

Further reading

Smith S, Scarth E, Sasada M. *Drugs in Anaesthesia and Intensive Care.* 4th ed. Oxford: Oxford University Press; 2011.

17A: False
17B: False
17C: False
17D: False
17E: True

Cell membranes consist of a phospholipid bilayer, through which most drugs need to pass to reach their site of action. There are a number of mechanisms by which drugs can cross the cell membrane, the most common of which is passive diffusion. Smaller molecules usually diffuse more readily, described by Graham's law, whereby the rate of diffusion is inversely proportional to the square root of their molecular weight. Phospholipid bilayers are hydrophobic; therefore, lipid-soluble drugs diffuse more readily across them. In addition, ionized fractions of drugs are repelled by the phospholipid bilayer.

Drug molecules move down a concentration gradient from areas of higher drug concentration to areas of lower concentration; Fick's law states that the rate of diffusion across a membrane is proportional to this concentration gradient. This is demonstrated by increasing the dose of the drug administered, thereby increasing the concentration gradient, to speed up onset of action. This effect is also demonstrated by Bowman's principle, whereby less potent neuromuscular blocking agents must be administered in a higher dose to exert their effect but consequently produce a larger concentration gradient and a more rapid onset of action.

Further reading

Peck TE, Hill SA, Williams M. *Pharmacology for Anaesthesia and Intensive Care.* 3rd ed. Cambridge: Cambridge University Press; 2008. Chapter 1, p. 1–7.

Roberts F, Freshwater-Turner D. Pharmacokinetics and anaesthesia. *Contin Educ Anaesth Crit Care Pain.* 2007; 7(1): 25–29.

18A: False
18B: False
18C: True
18D: True
18E: False

Not only does tobacco smoking result in many conditions that may require surgery, it also negatively affects outcomes from that surgery as well as the course of anaesthesia. Impaired oxygen carriage by haemoglobin, damage to the lungs and airway, as well as changes to the heart and circulation, can impair adequate oxygen delivery to tissues.

The long-term effects of smoking cessation, including reduction in chronic obstructive pulmonary disease and lung cancer, are well known; however, smoking cessation at any point prior to surgery can have beneficial effects on oxygen carriage and delivery, pulmonary function and capacity for physical work. Six months of abstinence from smoking can return pulmonary function to levels seen in non-smokers but before that time improvements in capacity for physical work can improve by 10–20% after just 12 hours; and upper airway irritability also begins to improve after this time with peak effects seen after 10 days' cessation. Smokers have higher levels (up to 10%) of carboxyhaemoglobin, which impairs oxygen carriage and delivery, but, as the half-life of carboxyhaemoglobin is 4–6 hours, even overnight abstinence prior to surgery can improve oxygen delivery.

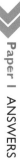
Further reading

Moppett I, Curran J. Smoking and the surgical patient. *Contin Educ Anaesth Crit Care Pain*. 2001; 1(4): 122–124.

19A: False
19B: True
19C: True
19D: True
19E: False

β-adrenoceptors are G-protein coupled receptors that include three varieties: $β_1$ receptors are found on cardiac myocytes and platelets, $β_2$ receptors in bronchial and vascular smooth muscle, and $β_3$ receptors on adipose tissue. β-adrenoceptor antagonists are used clinically in the management of hypertension and ischaemic heart disease as well as in the treatment of cardiac failure and for their anti-arrhythmic properties. There are competitive antagonists at β-adrenoceptors and some are more selective for a single subtype of receptor. For example, acebutalol has some $β_1$ selectivity, but atenolol, esmolol and metoprolol are more $β_1$-selective and therefore more cardioselective, with less unwanted side effects from $β_2$ receptor antagonism. $β_1$-adrenoceptors are G_s-coupled receptors whose activation leads to increased intracellular cAMP production leading to positive inotropic and chronotropic activity.

Propanolol and sotalol are both non-selective, binding to the $β_1$ and $β_2$ adrenoceptors. Some clinically available β-adrenoceptor antagonists are partial agonists. They exhibit agonist activity (sympathomimetic activity) in the absence of a full agonist but with limited intrinsic activity. In the presence of a full agonist, however, they act as competitive antagonists.

Further reading

Peck TE, Hill SA, Williams M. *Pharmacology for Anaesthesia and Intensive Care*. 3rd ed. Cambridge: Cambridge University Press; 2008. Chapter 13, p. 220–226.

20A: True
20B: True
20C: False
20D: False
20E: False

Thiazide diuretics such as bendroflumethiazide and metolazone act on the distal convoluted tubule to inhibit sodium and therefore water reabsorption from the tubule, producing diuresis. This increased sodium load in the distal convoluted tubule triggers simultaneous hydrogen ion and potassium excretion into the filtrate, which can lead to hypokalaemia and alkalosis. Hypokalaemia is also seen with loop diuretics, such as furosemide and bumetanide, but to a lesser extent. Loop diuretics act to impair the action of the counter-current mechanism within the loop of Henle by inhibiting sodium and chloride reabsorption.

Potassium-sparing diuretics, such as amiloride, block Na^+/K^+ ion exchange in the distal convoluted tubule, increasing sodium and therefore water excretion but preventing potassium excretion. Aldosterone antagonists such as spironolactone also act within the distal convoluted tubule, as well as at the collecting duct, but are competitive aldosterone antagonists, preventing reabsorption of sodium in the distal tubule and subsequent potassium excretion. Carbonic anhydrase inhibitors act at the proximal convoluted tubule to reduce the production of hydrogen ions from carbon dioxide and water, and therefore slightly increasing sodium and water excretion, which in turn stimulates potassium secretion.

Further reading

Clarke P, Simpson KH. Diuretics and renal tubular function. *Contin Educ Anaesth Crit Care Pain.* 2001; 1(4): 99–103.

Peck TE, Hill SA, Williams M. *Pharmacology for Anaesthesia and Intensive Care.* 3rd ed. Cambridge: Cambridge University Press; 2008. Chapter 21, p. 305–310.

21A: True
21B: True
21C: True
21D: False
21E: False

The Système International d'unités (SI units) were designed to produce a universally accepted standard for scientific measurement. The units are categorized into fundamental (or base), derived and supplementary units, although the supplementary units are not applicable to medicine.

There are seven fundamental SI units. These are the second, metre, mole, ampere, candela, kilogram and kelvin (remembered by the anagram SMMACKK).

From these fundamental SI units, several derived units are formed by combining one or more fundamental units by multiplication or division.

Unit	Symbol	Measurement	Definition
Derived Non-Electrical SI Units			
m^2	A	Area	Square metre
m^3	v	Volume	Cubic metre
$m \cdot s^{-1}$	S	Speed	Metre per second
$m \cdot s^{-1}$	v	Velocity	Metre per second in a given direction
$m \cdot s^{-2}$	a	Acceleration	Metre per second per second
Derived Electrical SI Units			
Volt	V	Electrical potential	I volt is the electrical potential between two points of a conductor, carrying a constant current of I ampere, when the power dissipated between these points is I watt. Voltage (V) = Power (W)/Current (I)
Ohm	Ω	Resistance	A conductor has a resistance of I Ω, when a potential difference of I volt applied across it produces a current of I ampere. Ohm's law, Resistance (R) = Voltage (V)/Current (I)

continued

Unit	Symbol	Measurement	Definition
Coulomb	Q	Charge	1 coulomb is the quantity of electrical charge transported past a point in a circuit in 1 second by a current of 1 ampere. Charge (Q) = Current (I) × Time (t). One coulomb is the charge carried in 6.24 × 10^{18} electrons.
Farad	C	Capacitance	A capacitor has 1 farad of capacitance if a potential difference of 1 volt is present across its plates when a charge of 1 coulomb is held by them. Capacitance (C) = Charge (Q)/ Voltage (V).
Units with Special Symbols			
Hertz	Hz	Frequency	1 hertz is one cycle per second (s^{-1})
Newton	N	Force	1 newton of force will give a mass of 1 kg an acceleration of 1 m·s^{-2} (kg·m·s^{-2})
Pascal	Pa	Pressure	1 pascal is the pressure exerted when 1 newton of force is applied over an area of 1 m^2 (N·m^{-2})
Joule	J	Energy	1 joule is the energy expended when point application of 1N force moves an object through 1 metre in the direction of which the force is applied (N·m)
Electronvolt	eV	Electromagnetic radiation	1 electron volt is the energy required to move 1 electron through a potential difference of 1 volt, in a vacuum. 1 electron volt is the equivalent of 1.6 × 10^{-19} J
Watt	W	Power	The rate of energy expenditure, where 1 watt = 1 joule of energy expended per second (J·s^{-1}).
Centigrade	°C	Temperature	1°C is equal in magnitude to 1 kelvin, however, 0°C = 273.15 kelvin.

Further reading

Clifton A, Armstrong S, Davis L. *Primary FRCA in a Box.* 1st ed. London: Royal Society of Medicine; 2007.

Cross M, Plunkett E. *Physics, Pharmacology and Physiology for Anaesthetists: Key Concepts for the FRCA.* Cambridge: Cambridge University Press; 2008. p. 18–21.

Marvel P. SI units and simple respiratory and cardiac mechanics. *Contin Educ Anaesth Crit Care Pain.* 2006; 6(5): 188–191.

22A: False
22B: True
22C: True
22D: True
22E: True

Humidity is the amount of water vapour present in a gas and can be described as absolute or relative.

Absolute humidity is the total mass of water vapour present in a given volume of gas (measured in mg·mL^{-1} or g·m^{-3}) NB the unit of volume is mL or m^3.

Relative humidity is the ratio of the amount of water vapour in a gas, compared with the mass of water required to saturate the gas at the same temperature. Relative humidity can be expressed as a ratio of the water vapour pressure compared with saturated vapour pressure (SVP):

Vapour pressure/SVP = RH (%) at that temperature

The dew point is the temperature at which the relative humidity of the gas exceeds 100% and water condenses out of its vapour phase to form a liquid (dew). The dew point is used to measure relative humidity using Regnault's hygrometer.

- Air at 100% relative humidity
  - At 20°C, the absolute humidity will be 17 $g \cdot m^{-3}$
  - At 37°C, the absolute humidity will be 44 $g \cdot m^{-3}$
- Air at 50% relative humidity:
  - At 50°C, the absolute humidity will be 44 $g \cdot m^{-3}$

Further reading

Wilkes AR. Humidification: its importance and delivery. *Contin Educ Anaesth Crit Care Pain.* 2001; 1(2): 40–43.

23A: True
23B: False
23C: True
23D: True
23E: True

Flow behaviour of a fluid (liquid or gas) can be determined by the density and viscosity of the fluid.

Viscosity is the property of a fluid that resists flow, or the 'stickiness' of a fluid. Increasing viscosity reduces flow; gases have a lower viscosity than liquids.

Consider laminar flow, which consists of parallel layers of fluid moving along a tube. Viscosity of the fluid is quantified by its coefficient of viscosity, which is determined by the shear stress and shear rate of the fluid as it flows along a tube.

- Shear stress is the force exerted on the fluid as it moves past a stationary object (drag). The velocity of fluid flow near the stationary object will be lower due to the shear stress exerted.
- Shear rate is the velocity gradient generated from the difference in velocity in different layers of fluid. This is a perpendicular gradient exerted from the most rapid to the slowest velocity vector.

The coefficient of viscosity (η) is calculated as:

$$\eta = \text{Shear stress/Shear rate}$$

The unit of viscosity is the poise.

Viscosity of fluid varies with temperature. In liquids, increasing temperature reduces viscosity. In gases, increasing temperature increases viscosity.

Newtonian fluids describe fluids where viscosity is constant, regardless of the velocity gradient (shear rate), for example, water.

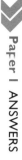
Non-Newtonian fluids may be shear thinning or rheotropic fluids.

- Shear thinning fluids: viscosity reduces as shear rate between the layers increases; for example, blood.
- Rheotropic fluids: viscosity increases with increased duration of the shearing force.

The Reynolds number is a dimensionless number that is used to predict whether flow will be turbulent or laminar in a given situation. Increasing viscosity reduces the Reynolds number, making laminar flow more likely when Re <2300; at Re >4000 inertial forces dominate making turbulent flow more likely. Note these calculations are based on flow in a straight pipe with uniform diameter.

Further reading

Smith T, Pinnock C, Lin T, Jones R. *Fundamentals of Anaesthesia*. 3rd ed. Cambridge: Cambridge University Press; 2009. p. 742–743.

24A: True
24B: False
24C: True
24D: False
24E: True

The Doppler effect is the phenomenon by which the frequency of transmitted sound is altered as it is reflected from a moving object.

This effect is used in clinical measurement to calculate the velocity at which a substance is moving. In the oesophageal Doppler, sound waves are emitted from a probe in the distal oesophagus at a frequency (F_O) and directed to the red blood cells in the descending aorta to calculate the *velocity* of blood flow. The sound waves are reflected from the moving red blood cells back to the probe at a new frequency (F_R), which is detected by the receiver in the probe. The difference between the emitted and received frequencies is the *phase shift* ($F_R - F_O$). This information can be used in the Doppler equation to determine the velocity of red blood cell movement in the descending aorta.

$$v = \frac{F_R \, c}{2 \, F_O \cos \theta}$$

where:
v = velocity
F_R = reflected frequency
F_O = emitted frequency
c = speed of sound in blood (1570 m·s⁻¹)
θ = reflected angle

If the cross-sectional area of the vessel is known (estimated using height, weight and gender), flow can be derived as area × velocity. This can be used to calculate cardiac output as the descending aorta typically receives 70% of the cardiac output.

The pressure gradient across cardiac valves is calculated in a similar manner, where velocity (v) is calculated using the Doppler equation and the Bernoulli principle is applied:

$$\text{Pressure gradient} = 4v^2$$

Further reading

Allsager CM, Swanevelder J. Measuring cardiac output. *Contin Educ Anaesth Crit Care Pain.* 2003; 3(1): 15–19.

25A: True
25B: False
25C: True
25D: False
25E: False
Be careful! The question is stating the definitions are *incorrect*, so the 'False' answers are, in reality, correct.

Force, power and work are derived SI units used commonly in anaesthesia to describe cardiac and respiratory mechanics.

Force (SI unit = newton) describes that which changes the state of movement or rest of an object. It is equal to mass (m) multiplied by acceleration (a).

$$F = m \times a$$

One newton is the force that will increase the velocity of one kilogram (mass) by one metre per second per second (acceleration).

Work (SI unit = joule) is the product of force (F) applied to an object and the distance (d) travelled in the direction of the force.

$$\text{Work} = F \times d$$

One joule is the work done when one newton of force is applied to an object to move it one metre in the direction of the force (N × m).

As work $- N \times m$, it can also be determined in terms of volume (m^3) and pressure ($N \cdot m^{-2}$):

$$m^3 \times N \cdot m^{-2} = N \cdot m^3 \cdot m^{-2}$$

$$= N \cdot m$$

Therefore, cardiac and respiratory work is considered in terms of change in volume multiplied by change in pressure.

Power is work done per unit time, and is represented by the watt, equal to one joule of energy per second.

Further reading

Marval P. SI units and simple respiratory and cardiac mechanics. *Contin Educ Anaesth Crit Care Pain.* 2006; 6(5): 188–191.

26A: False
26B: False
26C: True
26D: True
26E: False

Pulse oximetry was first introduced in the 1980s. It is considered a part of minimum monitoring standards and is an easy non-invasive method of monitoring patient oxygenation.

Components:

- Light-emitting diodes
  - Alternately emit light at two wavelengths: infrared (940 nm) and red (660 nm)
  - Off phase to allow for ambient light
- Photodetector
  - Detects transmitted light
- Microprocessor
  - Amplification and display

It uses two technologies:

- Pulse plethysmography: detects cyclical change in volume of artery with arterial pulsation. As volume increases, light absorption increases.
- Infrared spectroscopy: based on absorption of light by 'dye' in the tissues; namely, different haemoglobin species. Uses Beer–Lambert law:

$$A = \log_{10}(I_i/I_t) = \varepsilon LC$$

The Beer–Lambert law links absorption (A) of radiation to the:

- Intensity of the incident radiation (I_i)
- Non-absorbed element of the radiation (transmitted radiation I_t)
- Path length (L)
- Extinction coefficient (ε)
- Concentration of the absorbing substance (C)

The wavelengths of radiation used are those with differing absorption by oxygenated and de-oxygenated haemoglobin. At 660 nm, absorption of deoxygenated haemoglobin is greater than the absorption of oxygenated haemoglobin and at 940 nm, absorption of oxygenated haemoglobin exceeds that of deoxygenated haemoglobin.

Limitations of pulse oximeters:

- Accuracy decreases below 80% SpO_2
- Presence of other forms of haemoglobin which absorb light within the spectrums used
  - CarboxyHb: falsely high readings
  - MetHb: falsely low
  - Other dyes: methylene blue or indocyanine green
  - Not affected by foetal haemoglobin or bilirubin

- Movement and vibration artefact
- Electromagnetic interference: diathermy, mobile phones
- Hypertension or hypotension
- Vasoconstriction
- Hyperdynamic venous circulation (e.g. tricuspid regurgitation)

Further reading

Davey AJ, Diba A. *Ward's Anaesthetic Equipment.* 5th ed. Philadelphia: Elsevier
Saunders; 2005. Chapter 16, p. 350–352.

27A: True
27B: False
27C: False
27D: False
27E: True

Flow is defined as the quantity of fluid passing a point in unit time. Characteristics of fluid flow along a tube change when a constriction is encountered. The volume of flow rate is proportional to the area (A) of a tube and the average flow velocity (v) of the fluid. As a constriction is encountered, the area of the tube decreases and this is accompanied by a corresponding increase in velocity to maintain a constant flow rate:

$$A_1v_1 = A_2v_2$$

Bernoulli's principle applies the first law of thermodynamics, which states that the energy in a system cannot be destroyed or created but instead can change from one form to another. Bernoulli relates the pressure carried by the fluid as the potential energy and the velocity of fluid flow as the kinetic energy of the system. Bernoulli incorporates these principles in his equation for incompressible flow:

$$\tfrac{1}{2} \rho v^2 + P = \text{constant}$$

where
Kinetic energy = $\tfrac{1}{2} \rho v^2$ (ρ = density, v = velocity)
P = potential energy

The Venturi effect relates the Bernoulli principle to the flowing fluid as it encounters a constriction. It is the effect by which an introduction of a constriction to fluid flow within a tube causes the velocity of the fluid flow to increase and therefore the pressure of the fluid to fall. This effect allows the entrainment of another fluid substance, which moves along the pressure gradient that has been generated. Fixed performance oxygen masks, jet ventilators and nebulizers use the Venturi effect. The entrainment ratio is the ratio of entrained flow to driving flow.

Further reading

Smith T, Pinnock C, Lin T. *Fundamentals of Anaesthesia.* 3rd ed. Cambridge:
Cambridge University Press; 2009.

28A: False
28B: False
28C: True
28D: False
28E: False

The concept of flow of electric current can be confusing. In a circuit, current flows from positive to negative; however, this flow of charge is caused by the movement of electrons, which is in the opposite direction: negative to positive.

A parallel circuit has a number of circuit components arranged in a divided, parallel, manner. As the current flows from the electrical source, it will divide to flow along different branches of the circuit.

Resistors are used in a circuit to reduce currents and voltages; multiple resistors can be used. In a parallel circuit, the combined resistance can be calculated to calculate a total resistance (R_T):

$$1/R_T = 1/R_1 + 1/R_2$$

In a series circuit, the same current flows along the whole circuit without division. The total resistance is calculated by simple addition:

$$R_T = R_1 + R_2$$

Total capacitance (C_T) in a parallel circuit is calculated by simple addition:

$$C_T = C1 + C2$$

Total capacitance in a series circuit is calculated using the reciprocal:

$$1/C_T = 1/C_1 + 1/C_2$$

Current can be calculated, if the voltage and resistance is known, by using Ohm's law, which states that the current flowing through a resistance is proportional to the potential difference across it (effectively $V = IR$).

Further reading

Smith T, Pinnock C, Lin T. *Fundamentals of Anaesthesia*. 3rd ed. Cambridge: Cambridge University Press; 2009. p. 253–258.

29A: False
29B: False
29C: False
29D: False
29E: True

The Manley MP3 ventilator is a time-cycled pressure generator and a minute volume divider. It is composed of two sets of bellows: a smaller first set of bellows that receives the fresh gas flow and a second set, which is the larger, main set of bellows. There are three unidirectional valves: one between the two sets of bellows (the inlet valve), one between the second bellows and the patient (on the inspiratory limb), and the third between the patient and the adjustable pressure limiting (APL) valve (in the expiratory limb). There is an APL valve with tubing and a reservoir, which acts as a Mapleson D breathing system during spontaneous ventilation. There is a pressure gauge, an inspiratory time dial, a tidal volume adjuster, a control to switch from controlled to spontaneous ventilation and a rail to adjust the position of a weight that generates a pressure on the second bellows.

The ventilator is driven by the fresh gas flow that fills the first set of bellows on inspiration, while the second bellows is delivering its contents to the patient. The extent of the first bellows filling is determined by the inspiratory time valve. On expiration the first bellows empties its contents into the second bellows until a predetermined tidal volume is reached. In spontaneous ventilation, the system functions as a Mapleson D breathing system.

The Manley MP3 ventilator stops functioning early when there is a disconnection in fresh gas flow. The ventilator does not cope well with reduced lung compliance and the oxygen flush should not be used as it will cause barotrauma.

Further reading

Al-Shaikh B, Stacey S. *Essentials of Anaesthetic Equipment*. 2nd ed. Edinburgh: Churchill Livingstone; 2002.

30A: False
30B: True
30C: False
30D: True
30E: True
The Venturi effect describes the introduction of a constriction to fluid flow within a tube, causing the velocity of the fluid flow to increase and therefore the pressure of the fluid to fall. This effect can be used to entrain another substance, using both the pressure gradient and the viscous drag that has been generated by the flowing fluid. The entrainment ratio can be calculated as the ratio of the entrained flow to the driving flow. Venturi devices are used commonly in medical equipment. Examples are the fixed performance oxygen masks, nebulizers and jet ventilators. A further example of a device that works by the Venturi effect is the vacuum cleaner.

Further reading

Davis PD. *Basic Physics and Measurement in Anaesthesia*. 5th ed. Oxford: Butterworth-Heinemann; 2003.

31A: True
31B: True
31C: False
31D: True
31E: True

A defibrillator circuit consists of a capacitor, transformer, rectifier and an inductor. The transformer is a step-up component that increases the voltage from mains voltage (240 V) to around 5000–9000 V. This alternating current is converted to direct current using rectifiers. The rectifier contains diodes that allow the current to flow in one direction only. The defibrillator contains two circuits. The first circuit contains the components already described and shares a capacitor with the second (patient) circuit. Once the capacitor is charged, the circuit switches to the patient circuit. The patient circuit has paddles, which are connected to the patient to complete the circuit. The circuit also contains an inductor that allows the current, when delivered, to be maintained for several milliseconds.

Further reading

Singh S, Ingham R, Golding J. Basics of electricity for anaesthetists. *Contin Educ Anaesth Crit Care Pain.* 2011; 11(6): 224–228.

32A: False
32B: False
32C: True
32D: True
32E: True

In 1714, Fahrenheit used the mercury thermometer to develop his temperature scale. The zero point was set using a mixture of sodium chloride and ice. On this scale the boiling point of water is 212°F, the melting point of ice is 32°F and body temperature is assumed to be 100°F. It is the official temperature scale of the United States, Cayman Islands and Belize.

In 1742, Anders Celsius developed his scale. It is based on the properties of water: 100°C for the boiling point of water and 0°C for the melting point of ice.

The final scale by Lord Kelvin is the SI unit of temperature. The magnitude of one unit is the same as one degree on the Celsius scale. It is defined that zero kelvin is absolute zero. The kelvin is defined as equal to 1/273.16 of the absolute temperature of the triple point of water. The triple point is the temperature and pressure at which the solid, liquid and gas phase are in equilibrium.

Further reading

Sullivan G, Edmondson C. Heat and temperature. *Contin Educ Anaesth Crit Care Pain.* 2008; 8(3): 104–107.

33A: False
33B: True
33C: True
33D: False
33E: False

Gases are usually supplied from a central gas supply but each anaesthetic machine has its own backup supply in the form of cylinders. The cylinder has a valve block on the top of it. On it are marked the gas chemical symbol, tare weight, serial number and pressure at the last hydraulic test. Each cylinder is colour-coded for each gas or vapour. They are made from a molybdenum steel alloy, which is stronger and lighter than carbon steel. To prevent the wrong cylinder from being connected to the wrong yoke on the back of an anaesthetic machine, a pin index system is used. Situated between the cylinder and valve block is a plastic safety outlet that melts when heated to allow gas to escape in the case of a fire to reduce the chance of an explosion.

Further reading

Sinclair C, Thadsad M, Barker I. Modern anaesthetic machines. *Contin Educ Anaesth Crit Care Pain.* 2006; 6(2): 75–78.

34A: False
34B: False
34C: False
34D: True
34E: True
The voltage from a battery drives a steady current around a circuit. It does not vary in direction and so is termed direct current. In contrast, the UK mains electricity has an alternating current so that the voltage changes with time and the current changes direction back and forth. The voltage change follows a sinusoidal pattern. The number of cycles is termed the frequency and in mains electricity this occurs 50 times a second. Therefore, mains electricity has a frequency of 50 Hertz (Hz). Direct current does not change direction so has no frequency associated with it. The frequency of mains is chosen, as it is uneconomical to transmit electricity at high frequency long distances. It so happens that the risk of electrical shock is higher at these lower frequencies.

The voltage of mains electricity is 240V. This is not the maximum voltage level but is the root mean square. The maximum voltage is actually 340V. In transmission of electricity there is a loss associated with it. This is a product of the resistance of the transmission cable and the square of the current flowing through it. A standard electrical supply wire has three conductors within it: live, neutral and earth wires.

Further reading

Singh S, Ingham R, Golding J. Basics of electricity for anaesthetists. *Contin Educ Anaesth Crit Care Pain.* 2011; 11(6): 224–228.

35A: True
35B: False
35C: True
35D: True
35E: True

Medical equipment should be built to a British Standard. This standard classifies the equipment into three classes. This classification is based on the method of protection the equipment gives against electrical shock from the mains supply.

- Class I equipment: incorporates an earth wire, which has a low resistance so will cause an increase in current that will then melt a fuse breaking the circuit. The fuses are present in the live and neutral wire, and in the UK, in the mains plug too.
- Class II equipment: doubly insulated and does not require an earth wire.
- Class III equipment: has its own power source such as a battery and is not connected to the mains.

Medical equipment can also be classified according to the maximum permissible leakage current. This is either CF or BF. The F stands for floating and the C for cardiac. The floating refers to the added presence of a floating circuit.

- C equipment is suitable for connection to the heart as the current leakage is less than 50 μA. Type IIC has a maximum leakage of 10 μA and IC 50 μA.
- B equipment has a maximum permissible leakage current of up to 500 μA. IIB has a maximum leakage current of 100 μA and IB 500 μA.

Further reading

Davis PD, Kenny GN. *Basic Physics and Measurement in Anaesthesia*. Oxford: Butterworth-Heinemann; 2003.

36A: False
36B: False
36C: True
36D: False
36E: False

In biology the unit of percent (%) is used to denote the mass concentration of a solution. For example, 10 g of solute dissolved in 1000 ml of solution would be referred to as a 1% solution or 1% w/v (weight/volume). This is a slightly inaccurate way of expressing things and is frowned upon by pure chemists. It can be used in biology as the solute most commonly found is water based or aqueous. Therefore, 1000 ml of aqueous solvent would weigh 1000 g. Density does not affect things as biological systems are taken to operate at body temperature. The approximation also breaks down when very high solute concentrations are used where the density is changed but this is not physiologically relevant. Therefore, a typical 1% solution is taken as 1 g of solute dissolved in 100 ml of aqueous solvent.

Looking at the example in the question: 0.1 ml of solution would weigh 0.1 g or 100 mg. That is, 10 mg of lignocaine dissolved in this volume would then represent a 10% solution.

Further reading

Nic M, Jirat J, Kosata B. Mass concentration. *IUPAC Compendium of Chemical Terminology* (online ed.); 2006.

37A: False
37B: True
37C: True
37D: True
37E: False

Solids are classified as conductors, semi-conductors and insulators. This division is based on the solid's ability to conduct electrons. This ability is due to the presence of unpaired electrons in the outer shells of the solid's atoms. Most conductors are metallic, although the atomic structure of carbon in graphite allows it to act as a conductor. Insulators have firmly bound outer electrons such as rubber and glass, and will not allow an electrical current to flow. Semi-conductors under certain conditions, usually temperature, will allow an electrical current to flow. Examples include silicon, germanium, and gallium arsenide. Semi-conductors are used in thermistors, transistors and diodes. Electrical fuses are made of a metal wire and transformers consist of metal wire coiled around a ferromagnetic material.

Further reading

Singh SK, Ingham R, Golding JP. Basics of electricity for anaesthetists. *Contin Educ Anaesth Crit Care Pain.* 2011; 11(6): 224–228.

38A: False
38B: False
38C: False
38D: True
38E: True

Every cell has a membrane potential associated with it. This is due to the action of the Na^+/K^+-ATPase pump, which maintains a membrane potential of around 90 mV. Some tissues are able to depolarize, such as cardiac, muscle and neural tissue. These waves of depolarization can be detected by electrodes on the skin or connected to needles. Overlying tissues attenuate the magnitude of the depolarization. The potential of a single cell is 90 mV but what is measured at the skin in an ECG is around 1–2 mV due to attenuation. The potential of the EEG is much smaller: around 50 μV. The EMG has a much broader range of potentials due to differences in muscle size. The potential from a single motor neurone in an eye muscle will be around 100 μV but from a limb muscle it will be around 300 μV. This is because the motor neurone in the eye muscle supplies a few muscle fibres but in the leg it will supply a few hundred. The range of potentials in the EMG is from 10 μV to 10 mV: a 1000-fold difference. The duration of the EMG potential is much shorter than from an ECG, 5–10 ms compared to 1 s.

Further reading

Davis PD, Kenny GN. *Basic Physics and Measurement in Anaesthesia.* Oxford: Butterworth-Heinemann; 2003.

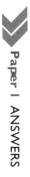
39A: False
39B: False
39C: False
39D: False
39E: True

Capacitance is the ability of a structure to store electrical charge. A capacitor consists of two conducting surfaces adjacent but separate to each other. A charge added to one surface induces an equal and opposite charge in the other. Capacitors are used in equipment such as defibrillators to store electrical charge and deliver high energy when required.

The smaller the distance between the two surfaces of a capacitor, the greater the capacitance between them.

$$\text{Capacitance (C)} = \text{Charge (Q)/Potential difference (V)}$$

The SI unit of capacitance is the farad.

As the potential across a capacitor rises, more energy is required to add the same amount of extra charge:

$$\text{Energy (E)} = \tfrac{1}{2}\ QV$$

These two equations can be amalgamated:

$$Q = CV, \text{ therefore } E = \tfrac{1}{2}\ CV^2$$

Further reading

Davey AJ, Diba A. *Ward's Anaesthetic Equipment*. 5th ed. Philadelphia: Elsevier Saunders; 2005. Chapter 2, p. 12–13.

40A: False
40B: False
40C: True
40D: False
40E: True

The thermodilution technique of cardiac output monitoring utilizes a pulmonary artery catheter to determine cardiac output. A known volume of cold saline is injected into the right atrium via the proximal port of the pulmonary artery catheter. A thermistor located in the tip of the catheter, which sits in the pulmonary artery, detects the change in temperature of blood flowing past the tip.

A computer then plots a curve of temperature over time. This curve can be changed to first demonstrate a decrease in temperature over time, and then a semi-logarithmic plot, from which the area under the curve can be used to determine cardiac output, using the Stewart–Hamilton equation. The numerator represents the mass of cold injectate, and the denominator represents the change in blood temperature over time.

$$\text{Flow} = \frac{V_{injectate}\left(T_b - T_i\right) \cdot K_1 \cdot K_2}{\text{Change in temperature of blood over time}}$$

$V_{injectate}$ = volume of injectate
T_b = temperature of blood at time 0
T_i = temperature of injectate at time 0
K_1 = density factor
K_2 = computation factor

Further reading

Allsager CM, Swanevelder J. Measuring cardiac output. *Contin Educ Anaesth Crit Care Pain*. 2003; 3(1): 15–19.

41A: False
41B: True
41C: False
41D: True
41E: False
Potassium is the predominant intracellular cation, with over 98% of physiological potassium stores being intracellular, mainly found within skeletal muscle. It is the second most abundant extracellular cation (after Na^+), and plays a major role in determining cell membrane potential, influenced by the Na^+/K^+-ATPase transmembrane transporter. Dietary potassium is absorbed from the small intestine and freely filtered at the glomerulus. Most potassium (90%) is reabsorbed in the proximal convoluted tubule and proximal loop of Henle. Active reabsorption or secretion of the remaining 10% occurs in the distal tubule and this controls potassium regulation.

Further reading

Clarke P, Simpson K. Diuretics and renal tubular function. *Contin Educ Anaesth Crit Care Pain*. 2001; 1(4): 99–103.

Parikh M, Webb ST. Cations: potassium, calcium and magnesium. *Contin Educ Anaesth Crit Care Pain*. 2012; 12(4): 195–198.

Tetzlaff JE, O'Hara JF, Walsh MT. Potassium and anaesthesia. *Can J Anaesth*. 1993; 40: 227–246.

42A: False
42B: True
42C: False
42D: True
42E: False

The human kidneys are paired organs situated in the retroperitoneum, which are responsible for urine formation, regulation of body water, sodium and other electrolyte balance as well as having an endocrine function. Each kidney contains over 1 million nephrons, which are the functional units of the kidney. The kidneys receive 20–25% of cardiac output at rest, receiving 500 ml per 100 g renal tissue per minute. This blood is filtered at the glomerulus producing 125 ml·min^{-1} of glomerular filtrate, totalling 180 L·day^{-1}. The glomerular filter consists of the glomerular basement membrane, the podocyte foot processes and capillary endothelial cells. Together they prevent the passage of large and negatively charged molecules. Twenty percent of the plasma entering the glomerulus is filtered into Bowman's capsule.

Further reading

Dwenger C. Renal morphology, blood supply and glomerular filtration. E-learning Anaesthesia Module 07b_19_01. Royal College of Anaesthetists. [Online] Available from http://www.e-lfh.org.uk/projects/ela/index.html.

Lote CJ. *Principles of Renal Physiology*. 5th ed. New York: Springer; 2012.

43A: True
43B: False
43C: True
43D: False
43E: True

Cardiac pacemaker cells and regular cardiac myocytes differ in the development of their action potential. Pacemaker cells, such as those found within the sino-atrial and atrioventricular nodes, spontaneously depolarize, conferring automaticity to the cardiac muscle. They do not have a stable resting membrane potential but the pacemaker potential gradually approaches a threshold due to decreased potassium permeability, a slow inward current of sodium ions and an associated voltage-gated increase in calcium influx via T-type calcium channels. Once threshold potential is reached, L-type calcium channels open leading to depolarization. Sympathetic stimulation to the heart decreases the potassium permeability of the pacemaker cells, increasing the rate at which threshold potential is reached. Ventricular myocytes, in contrast, do not spontaneously depolarize but have a stable resting membrane potential of approximately –90 mV. Following propagation of an action potential, voltage-gated sodium channels open and the resulting influx leads to depolarization. Following this, depolarization is potentiated by the opening of voltage-gated L-type calcium channels in the plateau phase. Activation of these L-type calcium channels is increased by catecholamines, reducing the plateau phase.

Further reading

Pinnell J, Turner S, Howell S. Cardiac muscle physiology. *Contin Educ Anaesth Crit Care Pain*. 2007; 7(3): 85–88.

44A: True
44B: False
44C: False
44D: False
44E: True

Pulmonary vascular resistance (PVR) is much lower than that of the systemic circulation (systemic vascular resistance: SVR), by a factor of approximately 10. In the absence of muscular arterioles (which control SVR), PVR is determined by a number of passive and active factors. With increasing cardiac output and consequent increase in pulmonary vascular pressures, PVR falls due to recruitment of previously collapsed capillaries and distension of the thin-walled pulmonary capillaries. Lung volume also impacts on PVR. The lowest resistance is found at FRC, whereas increasing lung volume increases the pulmonary vascular resistance by increasing transmural pressure across alveolar capillaries, despite increasing diameter of extra-alveolar vessels. Similarly, reducing lung volume increases PVR by reducing the calibre of extra-alveolar vessels, despite causing less collapse of capillaries.

Further reading

West JB. *Respiratory Physiology: The Essentials*. 8th ed. Philadelphia: Lippincott Williams & Wilkins; 2008.

45A: False
45B: True
45C: False
45D: False
45E: False

The Valsalva manoeuvre is performed by forced expiration against a closed glottis.

During this manoeuvre, a number of characteristic physiological changes occur, which demonstrate the reflex control of the circulation.

1. Increased intrathoracic pressure initially increases mean arterial pressure (MAP) by direct pressure effect on the aorta and by increasing venous return through the compression of pulmonary veins.
2. Increased intra-abdominal pressure thereafter reduces venous return by vena cava compression and therefore reduces MAP.
3. Baroreceptor reflexes act to increase systemic vascular resistance and heart rate, returning MAP to resting values.
4. Opening the glottis reduces intrathoracic pressure on aorta and reduces MAP. Initially blood fills pulmonary vessels and MAP remains low.
5. Baroreceptor reflexes again restore MAP.
6. As venous return now increases due to reduced intra-abdominal pressure, cardiac output increases but MAP overshoots due to persisting high systemic vascular resistance.
7. Increased stimulation of baroreceptors leads to reflex bradycardia and vasodilation and MAP is restored to normal values.

Further reading

Smith T, Pinnock C, Lin T. *Fundamentals of Anaesthesia*. 3rd ed. Cambridge: Cambridge University Press; 2009.

46A: False
46B: True
46C: False
46D: True
46E: True

Neurones are the main excitable cell type within the nervous system. They process and transmit information by the generation and propagation of action potentials.

Neurones consist of a cell body, a long projection called an axon, surrounded by supporting, non-excitable cells, and terminal buttons, which are found at the end of each of the branches originating from the axon.

Mammalian neurones have differing speeds of message transmission and different fibre lengths, and consequently transmit information governing different sensory modalities.

Nerve Fibres	Aα	Aβ	Aδ	Aγ	B (autonomic)	C	C (autonomic)
Sensation	Somatic motor, proprioception	Touch, pressure	Pain, temperature, touch	Muscle spindles	Preganglionic	Pain, temperature	Sympathetic postganglionic
Conduction speed (m·s⁻¹)	100	50	25	25	10	1	1
Diameter (μm)	10–20	5–10	2–5	2–5	3	1	1

Further reading

Cross M, Plunkett E. *Physics, Pharmacology and Physiology for Anaesthetists: Key Concepts for the FRCA*. Cambridge: Cambridge University Press; 2008.

Smith T, Pinnock C, Lin T. *Fundamentals of Anaesthesia*. 3rd ed. Cambridge: Cambridge University Press; 2009.

47A: False
47B: False
47C: True
47D: False
47E: False

Glucose, a six-carbon sugar, is the main transportable form of carbohydrate in the human body. The main 'energy currency' within the body is ATP, which can be generated by metabolism of glucose via the glycolytic pathway, the citric acid cycle and the process of oxidative phosphorylation.

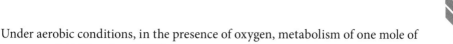

Under aerobic conditions, in the presence of oxygen, metabolism of one mole of glucose can yield 38 moles of ATP.

The first step in glucose metabolism is in the cytoplasm in the glycolytic pathway:

- Glucose is phosphorylated to glucose-6-phosphate.
- This is further metabolized, eventually resulting in 2 pyruvate molecules (a three-carbon molecule).
- Two molecules of ATP are used in the process.
- Four molecules of ATP are generated (net gain 2 ATP molecules).
- Two molecules of NADH; these can later generate more ATP by oxidative phosphorylation.
- The glycolytic pathway can generate pyruvate in the absence of oxygen.

In the presence of oxygen, glucose metabolism in the mitochondria begins when pyruvate is oxidized to acetyl coenzyme A (acetyl-CoA).

- Acetyl-CoA is the main entry point to the citric acid (or Krebs) cycle.
- The acetyl group (two-carbon) binds to oxaloacetate to create a six-carbon citrate.
- This passes around a cycle of intermediate carbon compounds until decarboxylated to regenerate oxaloacetate.
- Three NADH and one $FADH_2$ are produced in each cycle, which can enter oxidative phosphorylation.
- One guanosine triphosphate molecule is also produced.
- One glucose molecule can produce 2 pyruvate, therefore two cycles of citric acid cycle.

Oxidative phosphorylation takes place inside mitochondria:

- Electrons from the electron carriers NADH and $FADH_2$ are passed to a chain of electron carriers within the inner mitochondrial membrane.
- These electron carriers are a series of proton pumps, activated by the flow of electrons through them.
- They pump H^+ out of the inner mitochondrial membrane.
- H^+ moves back in along its concentration gradient through channels of ATP synthase, which catalyzes the generation of ATP.

Further reading

Nicholson G, Hall G. Diabetes and adult surgical inpatients. *Contin Educ Anaesth Crit Care Pain*. 2011; 11(6): 234–238.

48A: False
48B: False
48C: True
48D: True
48E: True

The brain has high metabolic activity, evidenced by its oxygen consumption and glucose utilization. Consequently, cerebral blood flow comprises 15% of cardiac output at rest, which equates to an average of 50 ml·100g^{-1}·min^{-1}. Metabolic differences between grey and white matter mean that they receive different blood flows: 25 ml·100g^{-1}·min^{-1} for white matter and 80 ml·100g^{-1}·min^{-1} for grey matter.

Control of cerebral blood flow is affected by many factors, many of which reflect the metabolic activity within the brain. Flow-metabolism coupling refers to regional increases in blood flow seen with increases in metabolic activity. As the cerebral metabolic rate for oxygen utilization increases, so does the cerebral blood flow. However, the increase in cerebral blood flow is more proportional to the increase in cerebral metabolic glucose utilization.

Cerebral autoregulation describes the maintenance of a constant cerebral blood flow (CBF) despite changes in cerebral perfusion pressure (CPP), by altering cerebral vascular resistance (CVR). The relationship between these factors is:

$$CBF = CPP/CVR$$

Autoregulation occurs between cerebral perfusion pressures of approximately 50 and 150 mmHg in the normal adult. Above and below these 'autoregulatory limits', cerebral blood flow increases or falls proportionally to cerebral perfusion pressure. In some individuals, for example those with hypertensive disease, these limits may be reset.

Cerebral blood flow is proportional to arterial partial pressure of carbon dioxide within the normal range. Below a limit of about 2.5 kPa, however, tissue hypoxia results in reflex vasodilatation, and a maximal level for cerebral blood flow may be reached at the other end of the spectrum. Arterial partial pressures of oxygen, however, only affect cerebral blood flow below a level of about 7 kPa, after which it is associated with significant increases in cerebral blood flow.

Further reading

Pattinson K, Wynne-Jones G, Imray C. Monitoring intracranial pressure, perfusion and metabolism. *Contin Educ Anaesth Crit Care Pain.* 2005; 5(4): 130–133.

Tameem A, Krowidi A. Cerebral physiology. *Contin Educ Anaesth Crit Care Pain.* 2013; 13(4): 113–118.

49A: False
49B: True
49C: True
49D: True
49E: False
Hydrochloric acid is produced by the parietal cells, which are located in the fundus and body of the stomach.

The following factors increase the release of acid:

- Gastrin
- Acetylcholine
- Vagal stimulation
- Distension of the body of the stomach
- Histamine

The following factors inhibit the release of acid:

- Acidity (negative feedback)
- Antimuscarinic agents
- Vagotomy
- Somatostatin
- Prostaglandin E_2
- H_2 receptor antagonists
- Proton pump inhibitors

The presence of acid helps to break down ingested proteins, activate pepsinogens, improve the solubility and hence absorption of calcium and iron and produce a toxic environment for pathogenic microorganisms.

Further reading

Jollife DM. Practical gastric physiology. *Contin Educ Anaesth Crit Care Pain.* 2009; 9(6): 173–177.

50A: True
50B: False
50C: True
50D: False
50E: True
In an adult the liver weighs approximately 1.5 to 2 kg. It is divided into lobes and the functional unit is known as the hepatic lobule. These are hexagonal in shape and have a central vein. In between the lobules lie the portal triad of a hepatic artery, portal vein and bile duct.

The central veins join to form the hepatic vein that drains into the inferior vena cava. The liver receives about 1.5 L·min^{-1} blood flow, which represents 25% of total cardiac output at rest. The liver accounts for 20% of the body's resting oxygen consumption. The liver's blood supply is dual, with 30% from the hepatic artery and the other 70% from the hepatic portal vein. The blood from the portal vein passes through the large and small intestines, spleen, stomach, pancreas and gall bladder. It is partially deoxygenated with an average haemoglobin oxygen saturation of around 85%. The portal vein contributes 50–60% of the total oxygen supply to the liver. The other 50% is from the hepatic artery.

Further reading

Peterson O. *Lecture Notes: Human Physiology.* 5th ed. Oxford: Wiley-Blackwell; 2006.

51A: False
51B: True
51C: True
51D: False
51E: False

The sympathetic nervous system is one component of the autonomic nervous system, the other being the parasympathetic nervous system. The two are different functionally, pharmacologically and anatomically.

The sympathetic outflow from the spinal cord takes place from preganglionic cell bodies located in the lateral horns of the spinal cord from T1 to L2. Between these two levels the anterior rami emerge together with white rami communicantes, which then enter the ganglia of the sympathetic chain. The chain in contrast runs from the base of the skull to the coccyx. It runs alongside the vertebral column about 2.5 cm from the midline.

Developmentally, there should be one ganglia for each spinal level but a number are fused. Typically there are 3 cervical, up to 12 thoracic, 2–4 lumbar and 4 sacral ganglia. The fusion of the lower cervical with the first thoracic ganglion is called the stellate ganglion.

As the outflow only occurs from T1 to L2, ganglia above or below these levels receive the preganglionic supply from axons ascending or descending in the chain. The preganglionic cells reaching the ganglia will synapse here, travel up or down a number of levels or pass through without synapsing and synapse in a peripheral ganglia; for example, coeliac, hypogastric and pelvic plexuses.

Further reading

Ellis H, Feldman S, Harrop-Griffiths W. *Anatomy for Anaesthetists*. 8th ed. Oxford: Wiley-Blackwell; 2003.

Whitaker RH, Borley NR. *Instant Anatomy*. 3rd ed. Oxford: Wiley-Blackwell; 2005.

52A: False
52B: True
52C: True
52D: False
52E: True

The bronchopulmonary segment is a discrete anatomical and functional unit. It is the smallest division of the lung that can be surgically resected without affecting the function of other lung units. There are 10 segments in the right lung and 8–10 in the left lung. A layer of connective tissue lies between segments giving a surgical plane for dissection.

Each bronchopulmonary segment is supplied by two arteries: a bronchial and a pulmonary artery that run through the centre of the segment. In contrast, venous and lymphatic drainage runs along the edge of the segment.

These are two mnemonics for remembering the individual segments:

Right lung: *A PALM Seed Makes Another Little Palm*

- Superior lobe
  - Apical
  - Posterior
  - Anterior

- Middle lobe
  - *Lateral*
  - *Medial*
- Inferior lobe
  - *Superior*
  - *Medial-basal*
  - *Anterior-basal*
  - *Lateral-basal*
  - *Posterior-basal*

Left lung: *AP ASIA ALP*

- Superior lobe
  - *Apico-Posterior* (merger of apical and posterior)
  - *Anterior*
- Lingula of superior lobe
  - *Superior lingular*
  - *Inferior lingular*
- Inferior lobe
  - *Apical* (or superior)
  - *Anteromedial basal* (merger of anterior-basal and medial-basal)
  - *Lateral-basal*
  - *Posterior-basal*

Further reading

Ellis H, Feldman S, Harrop-Griffiths W. *Anatomy for Anaesthetists*. 8th ed. Oxford: Wiley-Blackwell; 2003.

53A: False
53B: True
53C: False
53D: True
53E: False

The area of the globe anterior to the lens is filled with a clear fluid known as aqueous humour. It is produced by ciliary processes and flows into the anterior chamber through the pupil where it is absorbed into the trabecular meshwork into the canal of Schlemm.

The anterior chamber is the area posterior to the cornea and anterior to the iris. The posterior chamber is the area posterior to the iris and anterior to the lens.

The ciliary muscle is innervated by parasympathetic fibres that are transmitted via the occulomotor nerve. They synapse within the ciliary body and the postganglionic fibres reach the eyeball in the short ciliary nerves. When the ciliary muscle contracts, it pulls the suspensory ligaments forward and slackens them. The elastic lens becomes more convex and thus the refractive power is increased.

Further reading

Parness G, Underhill S. Regional anaesthesia for intraocular surgery. *Contin Educ Anaesth Crit Care Pain*. 2005; 5(3): 93–97.

54A: True
54B: False
54C: False
54D: True
54E: True

Two internal carotid arteries and two vertebral arteries supply the blood to the brain. These form an anastomosis called the circle of Willis. It is formed by the posterior cerebral, two posterior communicating, internal carotid, anterior cerebral and anterior communicating arteries. The anterior cerebral and middle cerebral arteries make up the anterior circulation.

The posterior cerebral arteries make up the posterior circulation and are formed by the division of the basilar artery, which is in turn formed by the fusion of the two vertebral arteries. Generally, each of the cerebral arteries supplies a surface and a pole of the brain. The anterior cerebral arteries supply the medial and superior surfaces and the anterior pole. The middle cerebral arteries supply the lateral surface and temporal pole of the brain. The posterior cerebral arteries supply the inferior surface and the occipital pole.

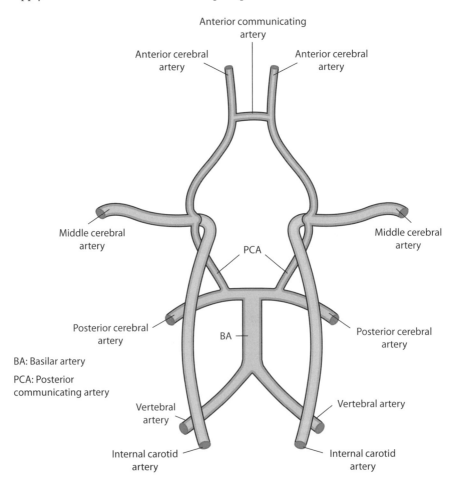

Further reading

Moore KL. *Clinically Orientated Anatomy*. Philadelphia: Lippincott Williams & Wilkins; 2009.

55A: False
55B: True
55C: False
55D: False
55E: True

Surfactant is produced by type 2 alveolar cells and stored in lamellar bodies before being released into alveoli where it sits between water molecules and reduces surface tension. Surfactant is composed predominantly of the phospholipids dipalmitoyl phosphatidylcholine and phosphatidylglycerol. Surfactant increases pulmonary compliance, stabilizes alveoli, reduces the transudation of fluid into alveoli and reduces energy expenditure as heat during respiration. Surfactant has a greater stabilizing effect on smaller alveoli.

Further reading

West JB. *Respiratory Physiology: The Essentials*. 8th ed. Philadelphia: Lippincott Williams & Wilkins; 2008.

56A: False
56B: True
56C: False
56D: False
56E: True

The kidney maintains an acid–base balance by three main mechanisms:

1. Secretion of H^+ and reabsorption of HCO_3^-
2. Excretion of titratable acid
3. Excretion of ammonia and ammonium

Secretion of H^+ and reabsorption of HCO_3^- occurs predominantly in the proximal convoluted tubule. Bicarbonate is freely filtered at the glomerulus and combines with hydrogen ions in the tubular fluid to form carbonic acid (H_2CO_3). Luminal carbonic anhydrase catalyzes the conversion of carbonic acid to carbon dioxide and water, which diffuse into the cell, where they are converted back into bicarbonate and hydrogen by intracellular carbonic anhydrase. The bicarbonate passes out of the cell into the plasma in exchange for chloride. The hydrogen ion is secreted into the tubule in exchange for sodium, where it binds with another bicarbonate ion. Intercalated cells in the distal tubule secrete hydrogen ions into the fluid. This is an active process as there is a considerable concentration gradient by this point. This occurs in conjunction with potassium and is under some influence of aldosterone.

In addition, hydrogen ions bind to filtered buffers in the urine and are excreted as titratable acid. The buffers are predominantly phosphate but beta hydroxybutyrate, creatinine and sulphates also contribute. The proximal tubule is the major site for this.

Glutamine is deaminated to form two ammonium compounds (NH_4^+) and two bicarbonate molecules in the tubular cell. The ammonium passes out of the cell (using the H^+/Na^+ antiporter) and is excreted in the urine. The bicarbonate is reabsorbed and enters the plasma. In addition, ammonia diffuses out of the plasma through the tubular cell and enters the urine, where it binds with a hydrogen ion to become NH_4^+. As this ammonium is a charged compound, it cannot diffuse back into the cell and is excreted in the urine.

Further reading

Chawla C, Drummond G. Water, strong ions, and weak ions. *Contin Educ Anaesth Crit Care Pain.* 2008; 8(3): 108–112.

Kitching AJ, Edge CJ. Acid-base balance: a review of normal physiology. *Contin Educ Anaesth Crit Care Pain.* 2002; 2(1): 3–6.

57A: True
57B: False
57C: True
57D: False
57E: True

Cellular respiration involves the oxidation of fuel molecules to generate adenosine triphosphate (ATP). Aerobic metabolism of 1 glucose molecule yields 38 molecules of ATP, however, this is only 40% of the total energy produced (60% is heat energy). The chain of reactions comprising aerobic metabolism of glucose begins in the cytoplasm with glycolysis, generating pyruvate, which is converted into acetyl coenzyme A (acetyl-CoA). Acetyl-CoA enters the mitochondrion and combines with oxaloacetate to form citric acid in the Krebs cycle (also known as the 'citric acid cycle'). The Krebs cycle takes place on the inner mitochondrial membrane and produces NADH and $FADH_2$, which act as reducing agents in the electron transport chain in the process of oxidative phosphorylation. The Pasteur point is the PO_2 threshold below which oxidative phosphorylation cannot occur; aerobic metabolism continues until the mitochondrial PO_2 falls below 0.4 kPa (3 mmHg).

Further reading

Burton D, Nicholson G, Hall G. Endocrine and metabolic response to surgery. *Contin Educ Anaesth Crit Care Pain.* 2004; 4(5): 144–147.

Power I, Kam P. *Principles of Physiology for the Anaesthetist.* 2nd ed. London: Hodder Arnold; 2008.

58A: False
58B: True
58C: False
58D: True
58E: True

Cholinergic receptors are either nicotinic (pentameric ion channels) or muscarinic (G-protein-coupled) receptors.

There are five subtypes of muscarinic receptors, of which M1, M2 and M3 are the most important.

- M1 is a G_q-protein coupled receptor that is found in autonomic ganglia and gastric parietal cells. Stimulation of the M1 receptor causes activation of phospholipase C, resulting in reduced membrane potassium conductance and depolarization of the membrane.
- M2 is a G_i-protein coupled receptor found in atrial tissue, in the SA and AV nodes. Activation reduces intracellular cAMP and increases membrane potassium conductance, hyperpolarizing the membrane.
- M3 is a G_q-protein coupled receptor that is found in glands and visceral smooth muscle.

Further reading

Power I, Kam P. *Principles of Physiology for the Anaesthetist*. 2nd ed. London: Hodder Arnold; 2008.

Smith T, Pinnock C, Lin T. *Fundamentals of Anaesthesia*. 3rd ed. Cambridge: Cambridge University Press; 2009. p. 253–258.

59A: False
59B: True
59C: False
59D: False
59E: True

For the sake of brevity, Arabic numbers rather than Roman numerals have been used in the explanation for this question.

The classical coagulation cascade has extrinsic, intrinsic and final common pathways, which culminate in the production of fibrin.

Tissue factor is the main activator of coagulation and forms the onset of the extrinsic pathway of coagulation. Tissue factor is a protein present in smooth muscle cells, fibroblasts and in the connective tissue matrix surrounding blood vessels. Injury to the vessel wall exposes tissue factor to circulating clotting factor 7, which binds to tissue factor and becomes activated to factor 7a Circulating factor 10 encounters the tissue factor/factor 7a complex and becomes activated to factor 10a.

Factor 10a cleaves prothrombin (factor 2) to release thrombin (factor 2a). The amount of thrombin produced is insufficient to activate fibrinogen at this stage. The thrombin produced instead activates platelets (primary haemostasis) and factor 5 (cleaves further prothrombin to thrombin). Thrombin also activates factors 8 and 11 (which in turn activates factor 9), in the intrinsic pathway of coagulation, where further factor 10 is activated, resulting in the generation of more thrombin.

When sufficient thrombin is produced, fibrinogen is cleaved to form fibrin and fibrinogen degradation products. Fibrin forms a cross linked matrix within the platelet plug to secure haemostasis at the site of injury.

Calcium is a cofactor in the activation of factors 9, 10 and 13 and in the cleavage of prothrombin to thrombin.

Further reading

Bombeli S, Spahn DR. Updates in perioperative coagulation: physiology and management of thromboembolism and haemorrhage. *Br J Anaesth.* 2004; 93(2): 275–287.

Smith T, Pinnock C, Lin T. *Fundamentals of Anaesthesia.* 3rd ed. Cambridge: Cambridge University Press; 2009. p. 253–258.

60A: True
60B: True
60C: False
60D: False
60E: True

A hormone is a chemical messenger, which exerts its effects distal to its site of release. At the target cell, a hormone binds to a specific receptor to produce a response. The receptor may be membrane bound or intracellular.

Membrane-Bound Receptors

Tyrosine kinase coupled

Membrane-bound receptor with an extracellular domain for ligand binding and an intracellular domain, which is coupled with enzymes. Activation of tyrosine kinase catalyzes a series of intracellular reactions. Examples are the growth hormone (GH), prolactin and insulin.

G-protein 3

Serpentine, membrane-bound proteins with an extracellular domain for ligand binding and an intracellular domain coupled with heterotrimeric G-proteins. Activation of the receptor triggers a cascade of intracellular reactions mediated by intracellular G-proteins. G-protein-coupled receptors are categorized into three types: G_s, G_i and G_q, according to the alpha subunit of the G-protein, which either stimulates or inhibits specific intracellular enzymes.

Examples include:

- G_s-protein-coupled receptor: oxytocin, antidiuretic hormone (ADH), leutinizing hormone (LH), follicular stimulating hormone (FSH), thyroid stimulating hormone (TSH), adrenocorticotrophic hormone (ACTH), adrenaline, parathyroid hormone (PTH), glucagon
- G_i-protein-coupled receptor: somatostatin, adrenaline (α_2-receptor), noradrenaline
- G_q-coupled receptor: adrenaline (α_1-receptor), ADH

Intracellular Receptors

Intracellular receptors act indirectly by altering DNA and RNA transcription and thus intracellular protein synthesis. These actions are slow in onset. Intracellular receptors are normally held in an inactive receptor form, bound with inhibitory proteins in the cytosol. Examples are steroid and thyroid hormones.

Further reading

Power I, Kam P. *Principles of Physiology for the Anaesthetist.* 2nd ed. London: Hodder Arnold; 2008.

1. **Magnesium sulphate:**
   A. Produces toxic effects that can be reversed by the administration of calcium
   B. Attenuates hypoxic pulmonary vasoconstriction
   C. Suppresses the response to laryngoscopy
   D. Has a diuretic effect
   E. Shortens the duration of neuromuscular blockade

2. **Propofol:**
   A. Is 3,6 di-isopropyl phenol
   B. Is highly protein-bound
   C. Has a high incidence of postoperative nausea and vomiting
   D. Has a pKa near physiological pH
   E. Is safe for use in prolonged high-dose infusions

3. **Thiopentone:**
   A. Is safe to use in porphyria
   B. Exists in keto form at physiological pH
   C. Is largely ionized at physiological pH
   D. Is presented in a glass ampoule in an atmosphere of carbon dioxide
   E. Is an oxybarbiturate

4. **The following drugs are correctly paired with the enzyme substrate that metabolizes them:**
   A. Midazolam and CYP 3A4
   B. Naproxen and CYP 1A2
   C. Omeprazole and CYP 2C19
   D. Sevoflurane and CYP 2D6
   E. Codeine and CYP 2E1

5. **The following pairings of drugs and effector sites are correct:**
   A. Aspirin: *COX-1*
   B. Dipyridamole: phosphodiesterase
   C. Ticlopidine: platelet surface ADP receptor
   D. Abciximab: glycoprotein IIb/IIIa receptor
   E. Clopidogrel: vitamin K epoxide reductase

6. Mannitol:
  A. Is presented as 1% and 2% solutions in 500 ml sterile water
  B. Has a tendency to crystallize at room temperature
  C. Has a high metabolic weight measured in daltons
  D. Has a bitter taste
  E. Solutions are acidic

7. Paracetamol toxicity:
  A. Causes thrombocytopenia
  B. Is less harmful in patients taking phenytoin
  C. Causes hepatotoxicity due to saturation of cytochrome P450 enzymes
  D. Is best treated with early administration of *N*-acetylcysteine
  E. Hepatic encephalopathy alone is an indication for liver transplant

8. The following agents are catecholamines:
  A. Dopamine
  B. Dobutamine
  C. Metaraminol
  D. Adrenaline
  E. Isoprenaline

9. The following antibiotics are bacteriostatic:
  A. Gentamicin
  B. Nitrofurantoin
  C. Erythromycin
  D. Doxycyline
  E. Metronidazole

10. Hartmann's solution:
  A. Is the same as lactated Ringer's solution
  B. Is also known as 'compound sodium lactate'
  C. Contains 111 mmol·L^{-1} of chloride ions
  D. Contains 154 mmol·L^{-1} of sodium ions
  E. Contains 4 mmol·L^{-1} of potassium ions

11. Morphine:
  A. Is an agonist at μ- and κ-opioid receptors
  B. Undergoes limited first-pass metabolism
  C. Is highly protein-bound
  D. Has a peak analgesic effect of 15–30 minutes after parenteral administration
  E. Has active metabolites

12. Sodium bicarbonate:
  A. May inactivate suxamethonium
  B. Can cause reduced tissue oxygenation
  C. Can be given orally
  D. Must always be given centrally
  E. Can cause arrhythmias

13. Anticonvulsants that act as voltage-gated sodium channels include:
A. Lamotrigine
B. Diazepam
C. Phenytoin
D. Sodium valproate
E. Carbamazepine

14. Hydrocortisone:
A. Is four times as potent as prednisolone
B. Acts on cytoplasmic receptors
C. Is less active than cortisone
D. Increases the risk of peptic ulcer disease
E. Can cause hypokalaemia

15. Oxygen toxicity is associated with:
A. Retrolental fibroplasia
B. Tracheobronchial irritation
C. The Paul-Burt effect
D. Pulmonary atelectasis
E. Anaemia

16. Sugammadex:
A. Is a cyclo-oxygenase compound
B. Has a hydrophilic core
C. Binds irreversibly to rocuronium
D. Is excreted unchanged in urine
E. Has an elimination half-life of 4 hours

17. Minimum alveolar concentration (MAC):
A. Is the concentration of intravenous anaesthetic agent required for 50% of patients not to respond to a standard surgical stimulus
B. Is decreased by pyrexia
C. Is decreased in neonates
D. Is additive if more than one volatile agent is used
E. Is increased by lithium

18. The following drugs exhibit affinity and intrinsic activity at μ-opioid receptors:
A. Nalorphine
B. Pentazocine
C. Nalbuphine
D. Buprenorphine
E. Morphine

19. The following inhalational anaesthetic agents cause an increase in heart rate:
A. Sevoflurane
B. Isoflurane
C. Desflurane
D. Halothane
E. Enflurane

20. The following drugs readily cross the blood–brain barrier:
  A. Diamorphine
  B. Dopamine
  C. Atropine
  D. Atracurium
  E. Glycopyrrolate

21. The following statements about heat are correct:
  A. It is the measure of how hot or cold a substance is
  B. 1 calorie is the amount of heat required to increase the temperature of 1 kilogram of water by 1°C
  C. It is a form of energy that can be transferred from one substance to another
  D. The SI unit is the kelvin
  E. 1 kelvin is 1/273.15 of the thermodynamic triple point of nitrogen

22. The following devices measure absolute humidity:
  A. Wet and dry bulb hygrometer
  B. Regnault's hygrometer
  C. Mass spectrometry
  D. Hair hygrometer
  E. Heat and moisture exchanger

23. Laminar flow:
  A. The most important fluid factor determining laminar flow is the pressure gradient applied
  B. Is inversely proportional to the fourth power of the radius
  C. Is directly proportional to the fourth power of the diameter
  D. Has a higher velocity than turbulent flow
  E. Is rapid in a 14 gauge peripheral cannula due to its length

24. The following statements are correct regarding diathermy:
  A. The patient forms part of the circuit in bipolar diathermy
  B. Cutting mode uses a continuous high-energy sine wave
  C. Diathermy uses mains frequency current at high-current density to produce heat
  D. Bipolar diathermy produces a power output of 400 watts
  E. Bipolar diathermy uses a neutral, low-current density plate to complete the circuit

25. Workplace exposure limits in the United Kingdom:
  A. For anaesthetic gases are measured over 15 minutes
  B. For halothane is 50 ppm
  C. For nitrous oxide is 10 ppm
  D. For enflurane is 50 ppm
  E. For isoflurane is 100 ppm

26. Regarding pulmonary artery pressure:
A. It is measured from the proximal lumen of a pulmonary artery catheter
B. Pulmonary artery catheters can only be inserted via the subclavian or internal jugular veins
C. Pulmonary artery catheters are typically 110 cm in length in adults
D. Measurement is inaccurate in the presence of mitral insufficiency
E. Wedge pressure is a reliable estimate of right ventricular end diastolic pressure

27. Soda lime:
A. Contains 94% sodium hydroxide when fresh
B. Changes colour when the pH falls below 13.5
C. Granule size is 4–8 mesh
D. Produces 120 L of carbon dioxide for every 1 kg of soda lime
E. Is more rapidly exhausted when higher fresh gas flow rates are used

28. The following statements are correct regarding transformers:
A. A transformer consists of two coils wound around a former
B. Transformers are used to distribute electrical power supply from the national grid
C. If the secondary winding has a greater number of turns than the primary, the voltage will be stepped up
D. DC voltages can be stepped up or down using a transformer
E. Transformers can be used to isolate an entire operating theatre

29. Problems with the self-inflating bag and mask system are:
A. That it does not apply positive end-expiratory pressure (PEEP)
B. That gastric insufflation may occur
C. That there is no outlet for exhaled gases
D. That it only functions when connected to oxygen
E. That it requires specialist training to use

30. The oxygen supply failure alarm:
A. Should be more than 7 seconds in duration
B. Should be audible 7 metres from the anaesthetic machine
C. Should be greater than 60 decibels
D. Is powered by the oxygen supply at 4 bar, upstream from the flowmeters
E. Will malfunction if there is failure of the electrical supply

31. Which of the following statements are correct?
A. Evaporation occurs when the molecules of a liquid have sufficient energy to become a gas
B. Evaporation requires potential energy, known as the latent heat of vaporization
C. When a liquid is heated, its saturated vapour pressure (SVP) increases in a sigmoidal fashion
D. Boiling occurs at the temperature when SVP equals atmospheric pressure
E. Above its critical temperature, a substance exists as a gas

32. **Which of the following pairings are correct?**
  A. Resistance thermometer: metal wire's resistance increases linearly with temperature
  B. Thermistor: the Seebeck effect
  C. Tympanic thermometer: Boltzmann constant
  D. Thermocouple: constantan
  E. Thermistor: metal oxide semi-conductor

33. **The following statements about blood pressure measurement are correct:**
  A. Too small a cuff will overestimate blood pressure
  B. The cuff should be 20% wider than the radius of the part of the limb being used
  C. Palpation of the artery as the cuff is deflated gives an accurate reading of systolic pressure only
  D. The inflatable cuff used is called a Korotkoff cuff
  E. It is part of the AAGBI minimum standard of patient monitoring for general and regional anaesthesia only

34. **The following pressures are correct:**
  A. Medical air for an orthopaedic saw: 4 bar
  B. Emergency oxygen flush: 4 bar
  C. Maximum pressure in reservoir bag: 60 cmH$_2$O
  D. Maximum pressure when the Heidbrink valve is closed: 7.0 kPa
  E. Oxygen failure alarm sounds when O$_2$ pressure <200 kPa

35. **The following pairings concerning exponentials are correct:**
  A. Exponential decay: nitrogen washout on preoxygenation
  B. Positive exponential: bacterial growth
  C. Positive exponential: preoxygenation
  D. Time constant: time taken for process to finish had initial rate of change continued
  E. Time constant^{-1}: rate constant

36. **Concerning measurement systems:**
  A. The rise time is the time taken from a step increase to 90% of the output being displayed
  B. Precision is how well a measured variable conforms to its true value
  C. Drift reflects how a measured value changes with time
  D. An arterial pressure monitoring system demonstrates a second-order dynamic response
  E. A temperature probe demonstrates a zero-order dynamic response

37. **Standard atmospheric pressure at sea level is equivalent to:**
  A. 740 mmHg
  B. 740 torr
  C. 14.7 lb·in^{-2}
  D. 10.33 mH$_2$O
  E. 100 kPa

38. **When measuring the central tendency of data:**
   A. The median is preferred to the mean when the data is not symmetrical
   B. The mode is sensitive to the effect of outlying data points
   C. The mode is the only index when using nominal data
   D. The median cannot be used if there are even numbers of data points
   E. The range measures the variability, which is the interval between the highest and lowest values in the distribution

39. **For carbon dioxide absorbers used in anaesthetic breathing systems:**
   A. The main constituent of soda lime is sodium hydroxide
   B. Soda lime containing potassium hydroxide has a greater tendency to form carbon monoxide with CHF_2 containing volatile anaesthetics
   C. Optimum granule size is 4–8 mm
   D. Soda lime absorbs more carbon dioxide per 100 g than barium lime
   E. Zeolites may be added to reduce the water content

40. **With electrical current:**
   A. Direct current flows through a conductor in one direction at a variable rate
   B. Alternating current flows through a conductor at a fixed rate and changes direction periodically
   C. Impedance is the sum of all properties resisting alternating current flow
   D. Impedance = Voltage/Current
   E. Reactance is the opposition to direct current flow resulting from capacitance and inductance

41. **The following are catecholamines:**
   A. Dopamine
   B. Dobutamine
   C. Ephedrine
   D. Dopexamine
   E. Noradrenaline

42. **Regarding glomerular filtration:**
   A. Glomerular filtration rate is 180 ml·min^{-1}
   B. Filtration fraction is approximately 20%
   C. Single nephron glomerular filtration rate (SNGFR) is greatest in cortical nephrons
   D. Molecules smaller than 70 kDa in size are freely filtered at the glomerulus
   E. Endothelial cells filter molecules over 60 nm in size

43. **Magnesium:**
   A. Is the second most abundant cation in the body
   B. 50% of stored magnesium is found in soft tissue
   C. 5% is found in erythrocytes
   D. Is directly negatively inotropic at the myocardium
   E. Enhances the positive inotropic effect of adrenaline

44. Pulmonary blood flow (PBF):
A. Can be calculated using the Fick principle
B. Is greater at the apex in upright patients
C. Increases at the apex during exercise
D. In 'West zone 2' is determined by the arterio-venous pressure difference
E. Is determined by passive factors under normal conditions

45. The stretch reflex:
A. Is a polysynaptic reflex
B. Uses afferent input from the muscle spindle
C. Has an efferent limb containing γ-motor fibres
D. Maintains constant muscle fibre length
E. Has afferent fibres that synapse in the dorsal horn of the spinal cord

46. Regarding nerve conduction:
A. Resting membrane potential in a neurone is –90 mV
B. At rest, the inside of the nerve cell is more negative than the outside
C. Above threshold potential of +30 mV, an action potential is generated
D. Above threshold potential, voltage-gated calcium channels open
E. Repolarization occurs due to opening of potassium channels

47. Regarding the foetal circulation:
A. It is a shunt-dependent circulation
B. Blood in the umbilical vein is 80–90% saturated with oxygen
C. Oxygenated blood from the ductus venosus enters the hepatic circulation
D. Only 25% of cardiac output enters the high-resistance pulmonary circulation
E. The ductus arteriosus preferentially supplies oxygenated blood to the brain and heart

48. In brainstem reflexes:
A. The afferent limb of the pupillary light reflex is the occulomotor nerve
B. The efferent limb of the gag reflex is the vagus nerve
C. The caloric reflex involves the vagus and vestibulocochlear nerves
D. The cough reflex tests the vagus nerve
E. The efferent limb of the corneal reflex is the seventh cranial nerve

49. Regarding the control of breathing:
A. The peripheral chemoreceptors are located in the carotid and aortic bodies
B. Stimulation of the carotid and aortic receptors causes a breathing response
C. J-receptor impulses pass to the respiratory centre via the glossopharyngeal nerve
D. The peripheral chemoreceptors are the principal receptors for monitoring changes in arterial carbon dioxide tension
E. The central chemoreceptors are responsible for around 20% of the ventilator response to hypoxia

50. High altitude causes:
A. An increase in the concentration of 2,3-DPG
B. A necessary decrease in the oxygen content of arterial blood
C. An increase in the pulmonary arterial pressure
D. A change in the capillary density of some tissues
E. An increase in renal excretion of bicarbonate

51. The following statements about the sacrum are correct:
A. The promontory is the posterior and upper margin of the sacral vertebra
B. It is composed of five fused rudimentary vertebrae
C. The canal contains meninges down as far as the lower border of the fourth sacral vertebrae
D. It articulates with the ischia laterally
E. The base articulates with the coccyx

52. The following statements about the lumbar plexus are correct:
A. It is formed from the anterior rami of the upper four lumbar nerves
B. It is situated within the body of the quadratus lumborum muscle
C. The lateral cutaneous nerve is purely a sensory nerve
D. The genitofemoral nerve is purely a sensory nerve
E. The obturator nerve is the largest nerve of the lumbar plexus

53. The diaphragm:
A. Possesses four openings
B. Is pierced by the vena cava with the left phrenic nerve
C. Is pierced by lymphatic vessels through all openings
D. Is innervated from the third to fifth cervical nerve roots
E. Its right crus has a larger area of origin than the left crus

54. For the brachial plexus:
A. There are more trunks than cords
B. Each trunk gives rise to two divisions
C. The lateral pectoral nerve is formed from the nerve roots
D. The cords are named according to their relation to the axillary artery
E. The long thoracic nerve arises from the C5, C6, C7 nerve roots

55. The stress response to surgery results in increased levels of:
A. Insulin
B. Glucagon
C. Growth hormone
D. Renin
E. Aldosterone

56. The following statements are correct:
A. Hypocalcaemia hyperpolarizes excitable membranes
B. Action potentials are propagated in a saltatory manner in myelinated fibres
C. The Nernst potential for potassium is −90 mV
D. The plasma membrane is freely permeable to calcium
E. The Na^+/K^+-ATP dependent cell membrane pump makes the resting membrane potential smaller

57. **Fatty acid metabolism:**
    A. Uses the carnitine shuttle to move fatty acids across the cell membrane into the cytoplasm
    B. Has a higher energy yield than glucose metabolism
    C. Occurs predominantly in the mitochondrial matrix
    D. Involves beta oxidation
    E. Produces acetyl-CoA, which enters the citric acid cycle

58. **The following cranial nerves carry parasympathetic fibres:**
    A. Trochlear nerve
    B. Oculomotor nerve
    C. Optic nerve
    D. Glossopharyngeal nerve
    E. Facial nerve

59. **Haemolytic transfusion reaction is likely to occur when:**
    A. Group AB patients receive group B blood
    B. Group A blood is given to patients who possess the red cell B antigen
    C. Group B patients receive group AB blood
    D. Group B blood is given to patients who possess neither the A nor B red cell antigen
    E. Group O patients receive group O blood

60. **The following compounds are synthesized by the hypothalamus:**
    A. Antidiuretic hormone (ADH)
    B. Prolactin
    C. Dopamine
    D. Oxytocin
    E. Somatostatin

2

PAPER 2
ANSWERS

1A: True
1B: True
1C: True
1D: True
1E: False

Magnesium is the fourth most plentiful cation in the body (after sodium, potassium and calcium) and is an essential cofactor in hundreds of enzyme reactions. Magnesium is a physiological antagonist of calcium and is essential for the production of adenosine triphosphate (ATP), nucleic acids and proteins.

Magnesium sulphate has a variety of uses. It can be used as an anticonvulsant in the management of eclampsia, as a tocolytic in the management of preterm labour, to terminate torsades de pointes, as a bronchodilator in acute severe asthma, to reduce spasms associated with tetanus and in the management of autonomic hyperreflexia (associated with spinal cord injury). Magnesium sulphate has been used to suppress the response to laryngoscopy, particularly in obstetric patients. In addition, magnesium is used to correct hypomagnasaemic states.

Pharmacodynamic effects of magnesium sulphate are:

- Cardiovascular: vasodilation, bradycardia and prolongation of AV nodal delay; attenuation of vasoconstrictor and arrhythmogenic effects of adrenaline
- Respiratory: bronchodilation, attenuation of hypoxic pulmonary vasoconstriction
- Central nervous system: anticonvulsant
- Gastrointestinal: osmotic laxative
- Renal: vasodilation, diuretic
- Uterine: reduction in uterine tone, increased placental perfusion, neonatal hypotonia (crosses placenta)
- Others: prolongation of clotting time, inhibition of platelet aggregation

Side effects of magnesium sulphate therapy are warmth, flushing, nausea, headache, dizziness, somnolence, areflexia, cardiac conduction disturbance, muscle weakness and also cardiac arrest. The toxic effects can be reversed with calcium. Magnesium prolongs the duration of neuromuscular blockade by reduction of presynaptic release of acetylcholine and reduction of post-synaptic sensitivity to acetylcholine.

Further reading

Smith S, Scarth E, Sasada M. *Drugs in Anaesthesia and Intensive Care*. 4th ed. Oxford: Oxford University Press; 2011.

Watson VF, Vaughan RS. Magnesium and the anaesthetist. *Contin Educ Anaesth Crit Care Pain*. 2001; (1)1: 16–20.

2A: False
2B: True
2C: False
2D: False
2E: False

Propofol is an anaesthetic induction agent that is used for the induction and maintenance of anaesthesia, and for sedation during surgical procedures and in intensive care.

The chemical formula of propofol is 2,6 di-isopropyl phenol, it has a pKa of 11 and is prepared as a white oil in water emulsion with soybean oil, purified egg phosphatide and sodium hydroxide. Propofol is physically incompatible with atracurium.

Propofol is not safe for use in high-dose prolonged infusions due to the risk of propofol infusion syndrome. This is a syndrome of metabolic acidosis, rhabdomyolysis, hepatomegaly, hypertriglyceridaemia, renal and hepatic failure and is often fatal. Risk factors include high dose infusion over long periods (>4 mg·kg^{-1}·hr^{-1} for more than 24 hours) and glucocorticoid use.

Further reading

Otterspoor LC, Kalkman CJ, Cremer OL. Update on the propofol infusion syndrome in ICU management of patients with head injury. *Curr Opin Anaesthesiol*. 2008 Oct; 21(5): 544–551.

Schüttler J, Ihmsen H. Population pharmacokinetics of propofol: a multicenter study. *Anesthesiology*. 2000; 92(3): 727–738.

3A: False
3B: True
3C: False
3D: False
3E: False

Thiopentone is a thiobarbiturate used for the induction of general anaesthesia, the termination of status epilepticus and for intracranial pressure control in traumatic brain injury. Thiopentone exhibits tautomerism, a type of isomerism where the structure of the compound varies depending on the nature of the environment. Thiopentone has a pKa of 7.6, so at physiological pH, 60% of the administered thiopentone is present as the highly lipid-soluble unionized form. At physiological pH thiopentone is in the keto form.

The compound is rendered water soluble by preparation in alkali form. Thiopentone is presented as a hygroscopic yellow powder in a glass ampoule with

6% sodium carbonate in an atmosphere of nitrogen. When reconstituted with water, a solution of pH 10.5 is produced, with the thiopentone molecule as the water-soluble enol form. The alkalinity of the solution would be reduced if air or carbon dioxide were present, hence the nitrogen.

Thiopentone is absolutely contraindicated in porphyria.

Further reading

Raferty, S. Thiopentone. *Update in Anaesthesia*. [Online] 1998. Article 8. Available from: http://www.nda.ox.ac.uk/wfsa/html/u02/u02_010.htm#prep.

4A: True
4B: True
4C: True
4D: False
4E: False

The cytochrome P450 group of metabolizing enzymes is a large and diverse group. They are responsible for the majority of Phase I reactions, where a molecule is rendered water soluble by oxidation, reduction and hydrolysis. The substrates of CYP enzymes include metabolic intermediates such as lipids and steroidal hormones as well as drugs and other toxic chemicals. The CYP 450 family of enzymes has many variations, broadly classified into CYP 1, 2, 3 and 4 indicating the gene family. This is followed by a capital letter indicating the subfamily and then another numeral to indicate the individual enzyme and the gene encoding it. The following are the enzymes primarily involved in metabolizing drugs relevant to anaesthetists:

- CYP 1A: bupivacaine, cimetidine, imipramine, ondansetron, theophylline, naproxen, paracetamol
- CYP 2C: diazepam, diclofenac, metoprolol, omeprazole, phenobarbitone, thiopentone
- CYP 2D6: codeine, tramadol, ondansetron, imipramine
- CYP 2E1: sevoflurane, other halogenated volatiles
- CYP 3A4: lignocaine, fentanyl, propofol, midazolam

Further reading

Park GR. Drug metabolism. *Contin Educ Anaesth Crit Care Pain*. 2001; 1(6): 185–188.

5A: True
5B: True
5C: True
5D: True
5E: False

All of the listed drugs are antiplatelet agents. Aspirin acts primarily on the cyclo-oxygenase 1 enzyme (*COX-1*), causing irreversible inactivation of the enzyme for the lifespan of the platelet. *COX-1* is responsible for the production of thromboxane A2, a potent vasoconstrictor and stimulator of platelet aggregation. Aspirin is 50 to

100 times more effective at *COX-1* inhibition than *COX-2*. Thus, aspirin causes little anti-inflammatory effect at low doses.

Dipyridamole is a pyrimidopyrimidine derivative. It has antiplatelet and vasodilating properties. Its effects are mediated by a rise in intracellular cyclic AMP by phosphodiesterase inhibition. It also blocks the re-uptake of adenosine by platelets, endothelial cells and red blood cells.

Ticlopidine and clopidogrel are both thienopyridines. They act to stop platelet aggregation by the irreversible inhibition of the $P2Y_{12}$ ADP receptor on the platelet surface. Vitamin K epoxide reductase is the enzyme that is inhibited by warfarin.

Abciximab (whose trade name is ReoPro™) is a monoclonal antibody that is a GP IIb/IIIa receptor antibody. They block the final common pathway of platelet activation.

Further reading

Smart S, Aragola S, Hutton P. Antiplatelet agents and anaesthesia. *Contin Educ Anaesth Crit Care Pain.* 2007; 7(5): 157–161.

6A: False
6B: True
6C: False
6D: False
6E: True

Mannitol is a polyol. It is an isomer of sorbitol and a sugar alcohol. It tastes half as sweet as sucrose and is used to mask bitter tastes. It is a naturally occurring substance found in algae, mushrooms and in trees. It has a low molecular weight of 182 daltons. The molecular formula of mannitol is $C_6H_8(OH)_6$. The dalton is the unit of weight used in the measurement of small molecules such as proteins or starches. Mannitol is thus freely filtered in the renal tubules. It is presented as a sterile solution of either 10 or 20% in 500 ml water. The solutions are acidic with a pH of 6.3.

Further reading

Shakat H, Westwood MM, Mortimer A. Mannitol: a review of its clinical uses. *Contin Educ Anaesth Crit Care Pain.* 2012; 12(2): 82–85.

7A: True
7B: False
7C: False
7D: True
7E: False

Paracetamol toxicity is responsible for 30,000 hospital admissions and 345 deaths each year in the United Kingdom. Paracetamol metabolism results in the production of a reactive intermediary metabolite, *N*-acetyl-*p*-benzoquinone imine (NAPQI), which is then rapidly inactivated by conjugation with glutathione. In paracetamol overdose, hepatic glutathione stores become depleted, resulting in accumulation of NAPQI within the hepatocyte, which causes hepatocellular necrosis. Early administration of *N*-acetylcysteine (NAC) replenishes glutathione stores and prevents hepatocellular necrosis from occurring. Patients taking hepatic enzyme-inducing drugs (such as phenytoin, rifampicin and carbamazepine) produce more NAPQI, thus are at greater risk of hepatocellular necrosis in paracetamol overdose.

Clinical features of paracetamol toxicity are often delayed and appear 24 hours after ingestion of the overdose. Nausea, vomiting, anorexia and right upper quadrant pain correlate with the onset of liver failure. Deranged liver function, coagulopathy and thrombocytopenia occur, with metabolic acidosis. Clinical features worsen after 3 days, where severe hepatic failure causes encephalopathy, cerebral oedema, lactic acidosis and hypoglycaemia.

King's College Hospital criteria for liver transplant in paracetamol toxicity are:

- Metabolic acidosis with pH <7.3 after adequate fluid resuscitation or
- The occurrence of all 3 of the following criteria within a 24-hour period:
  - Grade 3 or 4 hepatic encephalopathy
  - Prothrombin time >100 seconds
  - Creatinine >300 µmol/L

Further reading

Dargan PI, Jones AL. Acetaminophen poisoning: an update for the intensivist. *Critical Care.* 2002; 6: 108–110.

Ward C, Sair M. Oral poisoning: an update. *Contin Educ Anaesth Crit Care Pain.* 2010; 10(1): 6–11.

8A: True
8B: True
8C: False
8D: True
8E: True

There are many ways to classify adrenoceptor agonists, such as by the mechanism of action (direct or indirect), the chemical composition (catecholamine or non-catecholamine) or whether the agent is naturally occurring or synthetic.

Direct adrenoceptor agonists have a high affinity and selectivity for the receptor and act by direct stimulation. Endogenous neurotransmitters (mainly noradrenaline) are not depleted. Examples of directly acting agents are adrenaline, noradrenaline, methoxamine, dopamine, salbutamol, metaraminol, phenylephrine, isoprenaline, dobutamine and dopexamine. Indirectly acting adrenoceptor agonists act by a combination of increasing release and reducing reuptake of endogenous noradrenaline from the presynaptic terminal. Examples of indirectly acting agents are ephedrine and cocaine. A major problem with indirectly acting agents is reduced effect with repeated administration due to tachyphylaxis, which occurs when endogenous neurotransmitter stores are depleted.

Catecholamine is the term used to describe a chemical formulation consisting of a benzene ring with an –OH group at C3 and C4 ('catechol') and an amine side chain at C1 ('amine'). Noradrenaline, adrenaline, dopexamine, dopamine, isoprenaline and dobutamine are catecholamines. Ephedrine, metaraminol and phenylephrine consist of a benzene ring with an amine side chain, thus are termed 'synthetic amines'.

The main naturally occurring adrenoceptor agonists are adrenaline, noradrenaline and dopamine; all other agents are synthetic.

Further reading

Bangash MN, Kong ML, Pearse RM. Use of inotropes and vasopressor agents in critically ill patients. *Br J Pharmacol.* 2012; 165(7): 2015–2033.

Peck TE, Hill S. *Pharmacology for Anaesthesia and Intensive Care.* 3rd ed. Cambridge: Cambridge University Press; 2008.

9A: False
9B: False
9C: True
9D: True
9E: False

A bactericidal agent is one that kills bacteria and can be a disinfectant, antiseptic or antibiotic. Bacteriostatic antibiotics slow the growth or reproduction of bacteria. They must work in concert with the immune system to remove bacteria. The distinction between antibiotic action is not always clear. Some antibiotics are bacteriostatic at low doses but become bactericidal at higher doses.

Examples of bacteriostatic antibiotics include: tetracycline, sulphonamides, macrolides, trimethoprim and chloramphenicol. Bactericidal antibiotics include: β-lactam antibiotics, aminoglycosides, nitrofurantoin and metronidazole.

Further reading

Peck TE, Hill SA, Williams M. *Pharmacology for Anaesthesia and Intensive Care.* 3rd ed. Cambridge: Cambridge University Press; 2009.

10A: False
10B: True
10C: True
10D: False
10E: False

Ringer's solution is named after Sydney Ringer, a British physician and physiologist. In the 1880s he found that to keep an isolated frog's heart beating longer it must be bathed in a solution containing sodium, potassium and calcium salts in specific proportions (like most scientific discoveries this was accidental, as his assistant, instead of using distilled water, used London tap water, which happened to contain calcium ions in the same concentration as blood). Alexis Hartmann then added lactate to the solution producing Hartmann's solution.

Hartmann's solution contains: Na^+ 131 mmol·L^{-1}; Cl$^-$ 111 mmol·L^{-1}; lactate 29 mmol·L^{-1}; K$^+$ 5 mmol·L^{-1}; Ca^{2+} 2 mmol·L^{-1}.

Lactated Ringer's solution contains: Na^+ 130 mmol·L^{-1}; Cl$^-$ 109 mmol·L^{-1}; lactate 28 mmol·L^{-1}; K$^+$ 4 mmol·L^{-1}; Ca^{2+} 1.5 mmol·L^{-1}.

Further reading

Lee JA. Sydney Ringer and Alexis Hartmann. *Anaesthesia*. 1981; 36(12): 1115–1121.

11A: True
11B: False
11C: False
11D: False
11E: True

Morphine is a naturally occurring phenanthrene derivative. It is an agonist at the μ- and κ-opioid receptors. The μ-receptor is named after morphine whereas the κ-receptor is named after ketocyclazine. Morphine undergoes significant first-pass metabolism (bioavailability of 15–50%) and is 20–40% bound to albumin. Due to low lipid solubility its peak analgesic effect occurs at 30–60 minutes following intravenous administration. There is a poor correlation between plasma levels and analgesic effect. It is metabolized by the liver to normorphine, morphine-6-glucoronide and morphine-3-glucoronide. Morphine-6-glucoronide retains analgesic effects whereas morphine-3-glucoronide affects arousal. These compounds are renally excreted.

Further reading

Trivedi M, Shaikh S, Gwinnut C. Pharmacology of opioids. *Update in Anaesthesia.* 2008 [Online] p. 118–114. Available from www.worldanaesthesia.org.

12A: True
12B: True
12C: True
12D: False
12E: True

Sodium bicarbonate is an inorganic salt. It is incompatible with calcium salts and can cause inactivation of suxamethonium and adrenaline. Common indications for use include metabolic acidosis, forced alkaline diuresis, hyperkalemia or tricyclic antidepressant overdose. Complications of administration are hypokalaemia, excessive sodium load, a decrease in ionized calcium potentially leading to dysrhythmias and left-shift of the haemoglobin–oxygen dissociation curve leading to reduced tissue oxygenation. Sodium bicarbonate can be given either orally as a tablet or as an intravenous infusion. Intravenous solutions may be 1.24% concentration, which is iso-osmolar, or hyperosmolar 8.4%, which should be given through a central vein.

Further reading

Waldmann C, Soni N, Rhodes A. *Oxford Desk Further Reading: Critical Care.* Oxford: Oxford University Press; 2008.

13A: True
13B: False
13C: True
13D: True
13E: True

Anticonvulsants are drugs used to treat seizures and they act in a variety of ways. A seizure can be defined as the clinical manifestation of an abnormal and excessive discharge of neurones; therefore, modulation of this neuronal discharge can be targeted by pharmacological methods.

Benzodiazepines are commonly used, particularly in the short-term termination of seizures. Gamma amino-butyric acid-A ($GABA_A$) receptors are one of the major inhibitory neurotransmitter pathways within the central nervous system. They are pentameric ligand-gated ion channels, forming a central ion pore, which allows chloride ion passage through the synaptic membrane leading to hyperpolarization and preventing transmission of further signals. The $GABA_A$ receptor has a benzodiazepine binding site on the α/γ interface and binding of benzodiazepines potentiates chloride ion conductance by the $GABA_A$ ion channel.

Other anticonvulsants target voltage-gated sodium channels involved in depolarization and propagation of the action potential. Phenytoin binds to and stabilizes inactivated voltage-gated sodium channels, preventing further action potential generation. It may also potentiate the action of GABA as above. Carbamazepine acts in a similar fashion, as does sodium valproate.

Sodium valproate stabilizes inactivated voltage-gated sodium channels but also stimulates central GABA-ergic central inhibitor neurotransmitter pathways. Lamotrigine acts on the presynaptic neuronal membrane and stabilizes inactive voltage-gated sodium channels, leading to a reduction in release of excitatory neurotransmitters.

Further reading

Gratrix AP, Enright SM. Epilepsy in anaesthesia and intensive care. *Contin Educ Anaesth Crit Care Pain.* 2005; 5(4): 118–121.

14A: False
14B: True
14C: False
14D: True
14E: True

Glucocorticoids are one of two types of steroid hormone produced by the adrenal cortex (*cortico*steroids; the other type being mineralocorticoids, such as aldosterone).

Glucocorticoids are produced by the zona fasciculata of the adrenal cortex and act via cytoplasmic receptors to influence the rate of cellular protein synthesis. They have actions on many physiological systems, including positive cardiac inotropy, vasoconstriction and central nervous system excitation as well as stimulating gluconeogenesis and inhibiting peripheral glucose utilization.

Hydrocortisone is the main endogenous glucocorticoid in humans, and can be administered exogenously both as a replacement for glucocorticoid deficiency and

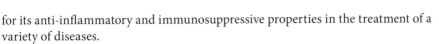

for its anti-inflammatory and immunosuppressive properties in the treatment of a variety of diseases.

If exogenous glucocorticoids are administered for long periods at high dose, it will suppress adrenal function by negative feedback on corticotrophin releasing hormone and ACTH. Therefore, the adrenal glands do not produce sufficient glucocorticoid in times of stress or after abrupt withdrawal of treatment. It must be supplemented in these patients peri-operatively to prevent hypotension, which can be severe enough to cause cardiovascular collapse.

- <10 mg prednisolone/day: not required as normal hypothalamic–pituitary axis
- >10 mg prednisolone/day: need supplementation

Hydrocortisone is a quarter as potent as prednisolone in its anti-inflammatory activity but has the advantage of parenteral routes of administration. Hydrocortisone also has weak mineralocorticoid effects, enhancing sodium and water retention and increasing glomerular filtration rate, as well as increasing potassium excretion in exchange for sodium, which can lead to hypokalaemia.

Further reading

Peck TE, Hill SA, Williams M. *Pharmacology for Anaesthesia and Intensive Care.* 3rd ed. Cambridge: Cambridge University Press; 2008.

Smith S, Scarth E, Sasada M. *Drugs in Anaesthesia and Intensive Care.* 4th ed. Oxford: Oxford University Press; 2011. p. 172–173.

15A: True
15B: True
15C: True
15D: True
15E: True

Oxygen is vital for aerobic metabolism, and the detrimental effects of acute hypoxia result in tissue damage and organ dysfunction. The benefits of supplemental oxygen in hypoxaemic patients are clear.

However, it may also be beneficial in some patients who are not hypoxaemic, for example, in the treatment of carbon monoxide poisoning, conservative resolution of pneumothorax and decompression sickness. In addition, supplemental oxygen is recommended to enhance oxygen delivery in critical illness to reduce organ dysfunction and improve survival.

Oxygen is a clear, colourless gas with a molecular weight of 32 and critical temperature of –118.4°C. It is available either in liquid form, stored in a vacuum-insulated evaporator or in cylinders of compressed oxygen gas at a pressure of 137 bar.

Hyperoxaemia carries its own risks, and should therefore be avoided in many cases. Oxygen can decrease ventilation due to a combination of reduced hypoxic ventilatory drive, ventilation–perfusion mismatch, reduction in vital capacity and absorption atelectasis. In a small population of susceptible patients who are dependent on hypoxic respiratory drive, this can precipitate hypercapnia.

Oxygen toxicity can also lead to formation of toxic free radicals, suppress red blood cell formation and cause retrolental fibroplasia in neonates.

Acute oxygen toxicity (the Paul-Burt effect) can occur with use of hyperbaric 100% oxygen and is characterized by altered mood, vertigo, convulsions and loss of consciousness.

Further reading

O'Driscoll BR, et al. Emergency oxygen use in adult patients. *Thorax.* 2008 Oct; 63(Suppl VI): vi1–vi73.

Smith S, Scarth E, Sasada M. *Drugs in Anaesthesia and Intensive Care.* 4th ed. Oxford: Oxford University Press; 2011. p. 264–265.

16A: False
16B: False
16C: True
16D: True
16E: False

Sugammadex is a cyclodextrin consisting of eight oligosaccharides arranged in a circular structure with a hollow core. Cyclodextrins have a hydrophilic outer surface but are lipophilic on their inner core. This allows them to irreversibly bind with lipophilic drugs, incorporating them within the core and eliminating them from plasma.

Sugammadex encapsulates free aminosteroid molecules (rocuronium, vecuronium or pancuronium) in the plasma and incorporates them into their toroid (doughnut-shaped) structure, where thermodynamic, van der Waals forces and charge transfer take place to irreversibly bind the drug. The muscle relaxant then moves from the neuromuscular junction down its concentration gradient back into the plasma, restoring muscle activity. Sugammadex has more affinity for rocuronium than the other aminosteroids.

The sugammadex-rocuronium complex is eliminated unchanged by the kidneys, with an elimination half-life of 2 hours.

It is administered as a single bolus intravenous dose; the dose given depends on the degree of residual block.

- T2 on train of four: 2 mg·kg^{-1}
- Deep block (post-tetanic count 1–4): 4–8 mg·kg^{-1}
- Shortly after administration for immediate reversal: 16 mg·kg^{-1}

Further reading

Khirwadkar R, Hunter JM. Neuromuscular physiology and pharmacology: an update. *Contin Educ Anaesth Crit Care Pain.* 2012; 12(5): 237–244.

Smith S, Scarth E, Sasada M. *Drugs in Anaesthesia and Intensive Care.* 4th ed. Oxford: Oxford University Press; 2011. p. 348–349.

17A: False
17B: False
17C: True
17D: True
17E: False

MAC is the concentration of volatile anaesthetic agent that prevents movement to a standard surgical stimulus in 50% of un-premedicated patients breathing oxygen at one atmosphere pressure. It is an indirect measure of potency of volatile anaesthetic agents, and is additive if more than one agent is used. MAC is decreased by concurrent use of sedatives, opioids and alcohol in the acute setting but is increased with chronic use. MAC is also decreased in the elderly and neonates, as well as in hypothermic or hypotensive patients and in pregnancy. Lithium decreases neurotransmitter release in excitable cells and inhibits brainstem catecholamine release, therefore decreasing MAC. Childhood and pyrexia increase MAC.

Further reading

Eger E. Age, minimum alveolar anesthetic concentration and minimum alveolar anesthetic concentration-awake. *Anesth Analg.* 2001; 93(4): 947–953.

Peck TE, Hill SA, Williams M. *Pharmacology for Anaesthesia and Intensive Care.* 3rd ed. Cambridge: Cambridge University Press; 2008. Chapter 8, p. 114–115, 278.

18A: False
18B: True
18C: False
18D: True
18E: True

Drug receptor interactions are commonly described in terms of affinity (how well a drug binds to a receptor) and efficacy or intrinsic activity (effect produced by the drug once bound).

An agonist is a compound that binds to a receptor to produce an effect. If this is a full or maximal effect, the intrinsic activity is said to be 1. A partial agonist is a compound that has an affinity for the receptor but is never able to produce a full or maximal response. It has intrinsic activity between 0 and 1.

Partial agonists exist at the opioid receptors but have limited clinical use. Nalorphine, pentazocine and nalbuphine show agonist activity at κ-opioid receptors but nalorphine and nalbuphine are antagonists at the μ-opioid receptor where they prevent binding of agonists. Buprenorphine has partial agonist activity at both μ-opioid and nociceptin receptors, whereas pentazocine also shows partial agonist activity at μ-receptors. Partial agonists can act as antagonists in the presence of a full agonist by preventing their binding and therefore reducing the maximal intrinsic activity achieved.

Further reading

McDonald J, Lambert DG. Opioid receptors. *Contin Educ Anaesth Crit Care Pain.* 2005; 5(1): 22–25.

19A: False
19B: True
19C: True
19D: False
19E: True

Sevoflurane is a polyfluorinated isopropyl methyl ether, which exhibits many of the properties of an ideal inhalational anaesthetic agent. It has a rapid onset of action due to its blood:gas partition coefficient of 0.7, and is relatively potent, with an oil:gas partition coefficient of 52. It has a minimum alveolar concentration of around 2%.

Unlike isoflurane, desflurane and enflurane, sevoflurane has a pleasant odour and is not an irritant to the upper airways and is therefore used for inhalational induction as well as maintenance of anaesthesia. Sevoflurane does, however, suppress respiration in a similar fashion to the other inhalational agents, reducing minute ventilation by a reduction in tidal volume despite some increase in respiratory rate.

All the halogenated inhalational anaesthetic agents lead to a dose-dependent reduction in systemic vascular resistance and an associated reduction in mean arterial pressure, despite the reflex tachycardia seen with isoflurane, enflurane and desflurane. Halothane in fact leads to a relative bradycardia. It has been suggested that isoflurane may cause 'coronary steal', preferentially dilating healthy coronary vessels and compounding ischaemia in diseased areas.

Sevoflurane has been shown to cause postoperative agitation in children on rapid emergence. Sevoflurane is 3–5% metabolized in the liver by the cytochrome P450 family of enzymes, by defluorination, producing inorganic fluoride ions, which are also produced by the metabolism of halothane (25% metabolized) and enflurane (2% metabolized).

Further reading

Young CJ, Apfelbaum JL. Inhalational anaesthetics: desflurane and sevoflurane. *J Clin Anesth.* 1995; 7(7): 564–577.

20A: True
20B: False
20C: True
20D: False
20E: False

The blood–brain barrier is a physiological and anatomical barrier separating the delicate and vulnerable tissues of the central nervous system from drugs and toxins present in the circulation. Tight junctions exist between capillary endothelial cells in contrast to fenestrations that usually make capillary membranes permeable. This prevents free movements of molecules across the barrier and most movement is by active transport or facilitated diffusion. Small, highly lipid soluble, unionized molecules may still pass by passive diffusion but large, highly ionized drugs such as non-depolarizing neuromuscular blocking agents are unable to pass. Similarly, in addition to the anatomical barrier, a physiological barrier also exists as part of the blood–brain barrier, whereby enzymes such as monoamine oxidase convert monoamines into inactive metabolites.

Further reading

Lawther BK, Kumar S, Krovvidi H. Blood–brain barrier. *Contin Educ Anaesth Crit Care Pain*. 2011; 11(4): 128–132.

Peck TE, Hill SA, Williams M. *Pharmacology for Anaesthesia and Intensive Care*. 3rd ed. Cambridge: Cambridge University Press; 2008. Chapter 1, p. 1–7.

21A: False
21B: False
21C: True
21D: False
21E: False

The difference between heat and temperature can be confusing, thus it can be helpful to revise the definitions.

Heat is a form of energy (measured in joules), which is possessed by the molecules within a substance. Heat energy will travel down a gradient from hotter to cooler substances (the second law of thermodynamics, i.e. a hot object will cool).

The SI unit of heat is the joule (as it is a form of energy).

Heat can also be measured in calories: 1 calorie is the amount of heat energy required to increase the temperature of 1 gram of water by 1°C (1 calorie = 4.16 J).

Temperature is a measure of the thermal state of an object in relation to the average kinetic energy of the atoms or molecules (how hot or cold it is, measured in degrees celsius or kelvin). For example, an iceberg has a low temperature but possesses a lot of heat energy due to the large number of molecules.

When heat energy is transferred to an object, the temperature of an object will increase.

The SI unit of temperature is the kelvin (K), where 1 K is 1/273.15 of the thermodynamic triple point of water

- 0°C = 273.15 K = 32 Fahrenheit
- 100°C – 373.15 K = 212 Fahrenheit

(Note: 1 K and 1°C are equal in magnitude.)

The specific heat capacity of an object is the amount of heat energy required to increase the temperature of 1 kg of a given object by 1°C. A substance with a large mass will require more heat energy to be applied in order to increase its temperature.

Further reading

Smith T, Pinnock C, Lin T. *Fundamentals of Anaesthesia*. 3rd ed. Cambridge: Cambridge University Press; 2009. p. 735–736.

Sullivan G, Edmondson C. Heat and temperature. *Contin Educ Anaesth Crit Care Pain*. 2008; 8(3): 104–107.

22A: False
22B: False
22C: True
22D: False
22E: False

Relative humidity is the ratio between the actual water vapour pressure in a sample of gas and the maximum water vapour pressure possible at that temperature (saturated water vapour pressure). Relative humidity is measured by the hair hygrometer, wet and dry bulb hygrometer and Regnault's hygrometer.

Absolute humidity is the mass of water vapour present per unit volume of gas (g·m⁻³). Absolute humidity can be measured using electrical means, chromatography, mass spectrometry and UV light absorption.

- Hair hygrometer: consists of a hair, stretched and attached to a spring, which is attached to a pointer on a dial. Increasing humidity stretches the hair and moves the pointer. The system is simple and accurate at relative humidity ranges of 30–90%.
- Wet and dry bulb hygrometer: consists of two thermometers—a 'dry' mercury thermometer, which reads the ambient temperature, and a 'wet' thermometer composed of a water soaked wick surrounding a bulb, which contains a thermometer. As the water evaporates, the loss of latent heat cools the thermometer until equilibrium is achieved. The rate of evaporation depends on the ambient humidity. The difference in the temperature between the wet and dry bulbs is recorded and relative humidity can be calculated using tables.
- Regnault's hygrometer: consists of a silver coated glass tube filled with ether. Air is bubbled through the ether, causing the ether to evaporate and cool. Condensation accumulates on the outside of the tube as the dew point is reached. Using the actual vapour pressure, the dew point and the SVP, the relative humidity can be calculated.

Further reading

Davis PD, Kenny GNC. *Basic Physics and Measurement in Anaesthesia*. 5th ed. Oxford: Butterworth-Heinemann; 2003.

Wilkes AR. Humidification: its importance and delivery. *Contin Educ Anaesth Crit Care Pain*. 2001; 1(2): 40–43.

23A: False
23B: False
23C: True
23D: False
23E: False

Flow is determined by:

- The pressure gradient applied, which is the driving force for flow
- Characteristics of the fluid flowing (viscosity, density)
- Characteristics of the vessel along which the fluid is flowing (length, radius)

Laminar flow is smooth, streamlined flow of low velocity. The fluid layers move in parallel, with lower velocity near the sides of the vessel due to shear stress (drag/friction) and more rapid movement in the centre of the vessel. The flow rate can be determined by the Hagen–Poiseuille equation:

$$Q = \frac{\pi \Delta P r^4}{8 \eta L}$$

where
  Q = flow
  ΔP = pressure gradient
  r = radius
  η = viscosity
  L   = length of the vessel

As the radius of the vessel is raised to the fourth power, this is the most important determinant of laminar flow. A 14G cannula is the most rapid due to its radius; although its length is longer, this factor is of lower importance.

Note that the Hagen–Poiseuille equation is also correctly described with diameter (d), rather than radius (r), hence d^4 instead of r^4. As diameter is twice the radius, the flow would be 2^4 times (16 times) higher, so this factor of 16 is applied to both the numerator (top of the fraction) and the denominator (bottom of the fraction), so 8 becomes $8 \times 16 = 128$. Hence the alternate equation is:

$$Q = \frac{\pi \Delta P d^4}{128 \eta L}$$

Further reading

Cross M, Plunkett E. *Physics, Pharmacology and Physiology for Anaesthetists: Key Concepts for the FRCA*. Cambridge: Cambridge University Press; 2008. p. 26.

Smith T, Pinnock C, Lin T. *Fundamentals of Anaesthesia*. 3rd ed. Cambridge: Cambridge University Press; 2009.

24A: False
24B: True
24C: False
24D: False
24E: False

Diathermy is a piece of electrosurgical equipment that is used for cutting, coagulation and securing haemostasis in a wide range of surgery. Diathermy works on the principle that a very high-frequency current (0.5–1.5 MHz) is passed to the patient over a high current density to produce heat. An alternating current is used, which has no adverse effects when used at these high-frequency ranges.

Diathermy may be monopolar or bipolar.

- Monopolar diathermy has two connections to the patient: the active electrode, with a high current density producing the desirable heating effects, and a neutral electrode, which forms a large flat plate with low current density completing the circuit. The patient forms part of the monopolar diathermy circuit, which has a high power output (400 W).

- Bipolar diathermy has two electrodes, both with high current density, often forming a forceps and the patient is not part of the circuit. Bipolar diathermy is of low power (40 W) so it is useful for smaller procedures.

Diathermy is available in two modes: cutting and coagulating. Cutting mode uses a continuous high energy, high-frequency alternating current to produce rapid heating over a small area. Coagulating mode uses bursts of current interrupted by periods of no current flow, resulting in local tissue heating with evaporation of intracellular water and dessication of cells resulting in haemostasis.

Further reading

Al Shaikh B, Stacey S. *Essentials of Anaesthetic Equipment*. 3rd ed. Edinburgh: Churchill Livingstone; 2006.

Boumphrey S, Langton JA. Electrical safety in the operating theatre. *Contin Educ Anaesth Crit Care Pain*. 2003; 3(1): 10–14.

Davis P, Kenny C. *Basic Physics and Measurement in Anaesthesia*. 5th ed. Oxford: Butterworth-Heinemann; 2003.

Smith T, Pinnock C, Lin T. *Fundamentals of Anaesthesia*. 3rd ed. Cambridge: Cambridge University Press; 2009.

25A: False
25B: False
25C: False
25D: True
25E: False

Exposure to substances in the workplace that may cause adverse health consequences are regulated in the United Kingdom by the Health and Safety Executive (HSE). They produce guidelines on workplace exposure limits (WELs) for such substances to minimize the likelihood of harm to the individual through exposure to hazardous substances. In the operating theatre, exposure to anaesthetic gases is regulated by measuring concentration in parts per million (ppm) of substances in the atmosphere within the theatre environment. They are averaged over a period of time, known as the time-weighted average. The time periods used are 15 minutes (short term) or 8 hours (long term).

Anaesthetic gas exposure limits are calculated over an 8-hour time-weighted average. The British WELs for anaesthetic gases are:

- Halothane: 10 ppm
- Isoflurane/enflurane: 50 ppm
- Nitrous oxide: 100 ppm

Further reading

Health and Safety Executive. *EH40/2005 Workplace Exposure Limits*. 2nd ed. Sudbury: HSE Books; 2011.

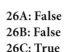

26A: False
26B: False
26C: True
26D: False
26E: False

Pulmonary artery flotation catheters consist of a multi-lumen catheter, 110 cm in length, and 7 or 7.5 French external diameter. They have a distal lumen, used for measurement of pulmonary artery pressure, with proximal lumens used for administration of various substances as well as central venous pressure measurement.

Pulmonary artery pressure measurement technique

- Catheter is inserted into internal jugular, subclavian or femoral vein
- Balloon is inflated with air and advanced
- Continual monitoring of pressure at distal lumen via pressure transducer
- Typical pressure variations allow for identification of right atrium, ventricle and pulmonary artery
- Catheter is advanced beyond the main pulmonary artery until wedged in branches to give pulmonary artery wedge pressure
- Balloon must then be deflated to prevent ischaemia

Pulmonary artery wedge pressure is used as an estimate of left ventricular end diastolic pressure.

At the tip of the pulmonary artery catheter a thermistor allows temperature measurement, allowing cardiac output monitoring by thermodilution techniques:

- Cold saline is injected via proximal port
- Temperature change as passes thermistor plotted as temperature over time curve
- Area under curve related to cardiac output calculated by the Stewart–Hamilton equation

Further reading

Davey AJ, Diba A. *Ward's Anaesthetic Equipment.* 5th ed. Philadelphia: Elsevier Saunders; 2005. Chapter 18, p. 369–371.

27A: False
27B: False
27C: True
27D: False
27E: False

Soda lime is used to prevent rebreathing of carbon dioxide in a circle breathing system, where low fresh gas flow rates are used. A combination of exothermic chemical reactions results in the absorption of CO_2 by soda lime, which is a granulated, hydrated lime. Soda lime consists of:

- $Ca(OH)_2$ (80%)
- NaOH (4%)

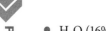

- H_2O (16%)
- Silicates (<1%, to bind granules)

Carbon dioxide reacts with soda lime by the following reactions:

$$CO_2 + 2NaOH \rightarrow Na_2CO_3 + H_2O + Heat$$

$$Na_2CO_3 + Ca(OH)_2 \rightarrow 2NaOH + CaCO_3$$

The pH of fresh soda lime is 13.5; when the pH falls below 10, the granules change colour. The standard granule size is 4–8 mesh (i.e. the particles can pass through a strainer with 4–8 openings per square inch), which is a balance between optimal surface area for absorption and minimal resistance to gas flow.

Problems with soda lime include the production of carbon monoxide when the CHF_2 group (a component of desflurane, isoflurane and enflurane) reacts with dry soda lime. Compound A is produced when soda lime reacts with sevoflurane, which has been found to be nephrotoxic in rats. Low fresh gas flow rates result in more rapid exhaustion of soda lime, as less gas is exhaled through the adjustable pressure limiting (APL) valve and more channelled through the soda lime canister.

Further reading

Al Shaikh B, Stacey S. *Essentials of Anaesthetic Equipment*. 3rd ed. Edinburgh: Churchill Livingstone; 2007.

Smith T, Pinnock C, Lin T. *Fundamentals of Anaesthesia*. 3rd ed. Cambridge: Cambridge University Press; 2009.

28A: True
28B: True
28C: True
28D: False
28E: True
A transformer consists of two inductors wound around the same former. Any current change in one circuit (the primary winding) will induce a current in the second coil (secondary winding) due to the coupling effect of the magnetic field generated. The degree of coupling depends on the number of turns in the primary winding, the secondary winding and the quality of the former. The greater the number of turns in the primary winding compared with the secondary winding, the larger the step down in the secondary circuit. This is used in the distribution of electrical power supply from the national grid and in the transfer of signals between circuits. In an operating theatre, transformers are used to isolate the operating theatre from the mains supply, producing a floating patient circuit that is not connected to earth. Transformers are used only with an alternating current.

Further reading

Boumphrey S, Langton JA. Electrical safety in the operating theatre. *Contin Educ Anaesth Crit Care Pain*. 2003; 3(1):10–14.

29A: True
29B: True
29C: False
29D: False
29E: False
The self-inflating bag and mask system is composed of a self-inflating bag with an oxygen reservoir and a one-way valve connected to a mask. The original system was developed in 1953 and sold through the company Ambu. As it was the first on the market, subsequent systems are often referred to as an 'Ambu Bag'. The valve has three ports: an inspiratory inlet through which the contents of the bag are passed to the patient, an expiratory outlet for exhaled gases and a connection for a facemask, endotracheal tube or supraglottic airway. The system is useful as ventilation can be achieved using air if there is no oxygen supply and it can be used by non-anaesthetists in emergencies. Problems with the system are that successful ventilation using a facemask requires a tight seal and gastric insufflation may occur. The system does not apply PEEP.

Further reading

Al Shaikh B, Stacey S. *Essentials of Anaesthetic Equipment*. 2nd ed. Edinburgh: Churchill Livingstone; 2002.

30A: True
30B: False
30C: True
30D: True
30E: False
The oxygen failure alarm requires no electrical power as it is powered by the oxygen supply at a pressure of 420 kPa, upstream from the flowmeters. Activation is thus pressure dependent, where a pressure-sensitive valve closes when the oxygen pressure falls to below 2 bar. The gas mixture is then vented, producing an audible warning tone that is greater than 60 dB, audible at a distance greater than one metre from the anaesthetic machine and of greater than 7 seconds duration. The same pressure-sensitive valve in addition opens an air entrainment valve and closes the anaesthetic cut-off valve to prevent a hypoxic gas mixture from being delivered to the patient.

Further reading

Al Shaikh B, Stacey S. *Essentials of Anaesthetic Equipment*. 2nd ed. Edinburgh: Churchill Livingstone; 2002.

31A: False
31B: False
31C: False
31D: True
31E: True
There is a unique temperature for a substance, called the critical temperature, above which the substance can only exist as a gas, irrespective of how much

pressure is applied to it. Below this temperature a substance can exist as a liquid or in a gaseous form, where it is called a vapour.

When a liquid evaporates, energy is required to overcome intermolecular bonds allowing the release of the molecules from the surface of the liquid into gaseous form. The energy invested is transferred from the liquid environment to the gaseous molecules, resulting in a drop in temperature of the remaining liquid. The energy is heat energy (rather than potential energy) and is known as the latent heat of vaporization. This concept explains why water vapour (steam) is more effective as a heating medium than hot water and is more hazardous. If the liquid is placed in a sealed container then equilibrium exists between the vapour above the liquid and the liquid. The pressure exerted by the vapour is the saturated vapour pressure (SVP). The SVP increases as the temperature of the liquid increases. The SVP increases with temperature in a non-linear fashion but not a sigmoidal one. When the SVP equals the atmospheric pressure the liquid boils.

Further reading

Boumphrey S, Marshall S. Understanding vaporizers. *Contin Educ Anaesth Crit Care Pain*. 2011; 11(6): 199–203.

32A: True
32B: False
32C: True
32D: True
32E: True
A thermometer is a device that measures temperature in a quantitative way. The different methods of measuring temperature are usually categorized into non-electrical and electrical.

Non-electrical systems rely on a change in the physical properties of a substance in relation to a change in temperature. To function reliably there needs to be a linear change in property related to temperature changes. Mercury expands in a linear fashion with an increase in temperature. It was incorporated into glass thermometers. They have a slow response time and have now been phased out due to the toxic nature of mercury. Alcohol can also be used in this way. It tends to give more reliable readings at lower temperatures as its boiling point is 78.5°C.

Electrical methods of temperature measurement include the resistance thermometer, thermistor, thermocouple and infrared tympanic thermometer.

- Resistance thermometer: the resistance of a metal wire increases linearly with temperature. The most common metal used is platinum and the wire is incorporated into a Wheatstone bridge.
- Thermistor: this uses a metal oxide semi-conductor. As the temperature increases, the resistance of the semi-conductor decreases exponentially. These devices are very accurate, can be made very small and are robust, although they do not tolerate extreme changes in temperature. This makes the thermistor ideal for measuring changes in body temperature.
- Thermocouple: this utilizes the Seebeck effect (Thomas Seebeck, a German-Estonian physicist, originally observed that a compass needle was deflected

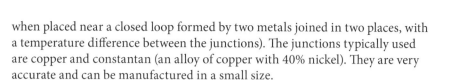

when placed near a closed loop formed by two metals joined in two places, with a temperature difference between the junctions). The junctions typically used are copper and constantan (an alloy of copper with 40% nickel). They are very accurate and can be manufactured in a small size.

- Infrared tympanic thermometer: this measures the infrared radiation emitted by the tympanic membrane. A thermopile is used in the device, which is a collection of thermocouples. This device relies on the Stefan–Boltzmann law, which states that as a body's temperature increases the amount of infrared radiation will also increase.

Further reading

Sullivan G, Edmondson C. Heat and temperature. *Contin Educ Anaesth Crit Care Pain.* 2008; 8(3): 104–107.

33A: True
33B: False
33C: False
33D: False
33E: False

The first sphygmomanometer (derived from the Greek for 'pulse', *sphygmos*, and *manometer*, a pressure meter), was supposedly invented by Riva Rocci, an Italian physician. The cuff is often called a Riva Rocci cuff. Korotkoff was a Russian who commented on the sounds heard during auscultation of the brachial artery during cuff deflation. Too small a cuff will overestimate blood pressure and too big will underestimate. The cuff should be 20% wider than the diameter of the part of the limb being used. Estimation of the systolic blood pressure by palpation of the artery can underestimate its true value by as much as 25%. The Association of Anaesthetists of Great Britain and Ireland (AAGBI) recommend that blood pressure measurement should also be used when patients are undergoing general anaesthesia, regional anaesthesia and sedation.

Further reading

Ward M, Langton J. Blood pressure measurement. *Contin Educ Anaesth Crit Care Pain.* 2007; 7(4): 122–126.

34A: False
34B: True
34C: True
34D: True
34E: True

Gases are supplied through the hospital pipeline at a pressure of 4 bar. The medical air used to power surgical instruments is at a higher pressure of 7.0 bar. The oxygen flush bypasses the back bar and supplies oxygen by high pressure directly at a flow rate of 37–75 L·min^{-1} and a pressure of 4 bar. The Heidbrink valve is the eponymous name for the adjustable pressure limiting (APL) valve. When in the open position it needs a pressure of less than 1 cmH$_2$O to open it, and when closed will need a pressure of 70 cmH$_2$O (or 7.0 kPa) to open it. The reservoir bag serves to protect the patient from barotrauma and has a maximal attainable pressure of 60 cmH$_2$O.

Further reading

Sinclair CM, Thadsad MK, Barker I. Modern anaesthetic machines. *Contin Educ Anaesth Crit Care Pain.* 2006; 6(2): 75–78.

35A: True
35B: True
35C: False
35D: True
35E: True

The exponential function is used to model a process in which a constant change in the independent variable gives the same proportional change in the dependent variable.

Examples of exponential processes include exponential decay such as radioactive decay, nitrogen washout and most drug elimination (a first-order process). An exponential build-up is an example of a wash-in process such as the inhalation of volatile anaesthetics, preoxygenation or lung inflation with pressure control ventilation. A positive exponential process occurs in the growth of a bacterial colony.

The exponential function can be defined by the half-life, which is the time taken for the quantity to decrease to 50% of its original value. The time constant (τ, tau) refers to the time that would be taken for the process to finish, had the initial rate of change continued. The reciprocal of the time constant is equal to the rate constant.

Further reading

Clifton B, Armstrong S, Davis L. *Primary FRCA in a Box.* London: RSM Books; 2007.

36A: False
36B: False
36C: True
36D: True
36E: False

Measurement systems act by converting a biological signal into a form that can be displayed and recorded. To be reliable the measurement system has to give repeatable results and must be able to be calibrated. Measurement systems are required to monitor both static signals and ones that are constantly changing (dynamic responses). How well a measured value conforms to its true value is called 'accuracy'. Precision reflects how well a system will repeatedly produce the same value. Drift reflects how well a measured value changes with time.

When there is a step change in the signal, the response of the measuring system can be described by the response and the rise time. The response time is the time from the step change in signal to 90% of the final output value being displayed. The rise time is the time taken from 10–90% of the output value being displayed.

Dynamic responses can be zero, first and second order. Zero-order responses track a signal exactly. First-order responses track the signal exponentially, for example, temperature probe warming up. Second-order responses may oscillate around the signal, for example, arterial blood pressure monitoring.

Further reading

Dolenska S. *Basic Science for Anaesthetists*. Cambridge: Cambridge University Press; 2006.

37A: False
37B: False
37C: True
37D: True
37E: False
The standard atmosphere (atm) is a unit of pressure. It is defined as being, at sea level: temperature 20°C, relative humidity 20%, and air density 1.225 kg/m^3. It has a number of equivalents.

1 atm is equal to: 760 torr, 760 mmHg, 14.7 psi (lb·in^{-2}), 10.33 mH$_2$O, 1013 millibars and 101.325 kPa.

The atmosphere is the pressure standard used by the petroleum and aerospace industry, and in pneumatic fluid power. In 1971 the International Union of Pure and Applied Chemistry (IUPAC) declared that a different standard should be used when determining the properties of substances and set the pressure standard at 100 kPa equivalent to 750.1 mmHg.

Further reading

Davis P, Kenny C. *Basic Physics and Measurement in Anaesthesia*. 5th ed. Oxford: Butterworth-Heinemann; 2003.

Ewing MB, et al. Standard quantities in chemical thermodynamics. Fugacities, activities and equilibrium constants for pure and mixed phases (IUPAC Recommendations 1994). *Pure and Appl Chem*. 1994; 66(3): 533.

38A: True
38B: False
38C: True
38D: False
38E: True
Central tendency refers to the way in which quantitative data tends to cluster around some value. A measure of central tendency is any way of specifying this central value. The three that are in most common usage are the mode, median and the mean.

The mode is simply the most common or popular value in the data set. It is the only measure available for use with nominal data, for example, most common name in a class or year group. It can also be used for ordinal or interval data but is less useful.

The median is the middle value if there are odd numbers of data points and the mean of the two middle values if there are even numbers of data points. The

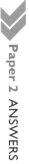

median is less affected by outlying data points so is more reflective of the central value in data that is not normally distributed.

The mean is the 'average' (the sum of values divided by the number of values) and is affected by outliers if the data is skewed in some way. It is the better measure of central tendency in a normal distribution.

Variability refers to the measurement of the spread of data.

Range is the interval between the highest and lowest values in the distribution. Interquartile range is the interval between the 25th percentile and the 75th percentile value.

Further reading

McCluskey A, Lalkhen AG. Statistics II: central tendency and spread of data. *Contin Educ Anaesth Crit Care Pain*. 2007; 7(4): 127–130.

39A: False
39B: True
39C: False
39D: False
39E: False

CO_2 must be removed from exhaled gases in order to allow low gas flows to be used without rebreathing of CO_2. This can be achieved using substances that absorb CO_2 during an exothermic reaction, which requires the presence of water.

Granules must be small enough to allow optimum surface area for absorption but large enough to prevent excess resistance to breathing. Usual size is 4–8 mesh (this means the granules will pass through a sieve with four strands per inch but not one with eight strands per inch).

The most commonly used absorbent is soda lime, the main constituent of which is calcium hydroxide.

Other constituents:

- Sodium (or potassium) hydroxide: added to enhance reactivity and ability to bind water
- Barium: used in barium lime with potassium hydroxide; no longer commercially available
- Zeolites: micropourous crystalline solids, which may be added to increase porosity, hardness and water content
- Silica
- Calcium chloride

Carbon dioxide reacts with soda lime by the following reactions:

$$CO_2 + 2NaOH \rightarrow Na_2CO_3 + H_2O + Heat$$

$$Na_2CO_3 + Ca(OH)_2 \rightarrow 2NaOH + CaCO_3$$

This reaction changes the pH of the soda lime; indicator dyes are added to show when the soda lime is used up.

Soda lime is capable of absorbing 25 litres of carbon dioxide per 100 g (barium lime 27 litres per 100 g).

Anaesthetic agents with CHF_2 (desflurane, enflurane and isoflurane) react with dry warm soda lime or barium lime to produce carbon monoxide. This is prevented by fresh soda lime but is greater in soda-lime-containing potassium rather than sodium hydroxide.

Further reading

Davey AJ, Diba A. *Ward's Anaesthetic Equipment*. 5th ed. Philadelphia: Elsevier Saunders; 2005. Chapter 7, p. 142–146.

40A: False
40B: False
40C: True
40D: True
40E: False

Electric current is the flow of electrically charged particles across a conducting material when an electric potential exists across it.

The SI unit of current is the ampere (A), which equals the current in two parallel conductors of infinite length placed 1 metre apart in a vacuum, which would produce between them a force of 2×10^{-7} N·m^{-1}. Also described as the flow of one coulomb of charge per second.

Current can be either direct current or alternating current, each of which has different properties.

Direct current (DC) is current that flows through a conductor in one direction at a fixed rate.

- When current flows through a resistance, a heating effect occurs (or power converted to other form of energy). This power (watts) can be calculated by $P = IV$, where I is the current in amperes, and V is the potential difference across the resistance.

Alternating current (AC) is current that flows through a conductor changing direction periodically.

- Its waveform may be any shape, and its value ranges throughout the cycle, so commonly it is described by the equivalent direct current value that would provide the same heating effect. This is known as the root mean square (RMS).
- $P = IV$ and $V = IR$, therefore $P = I^2R$.
- The flow of a variable current in a circuit produces reactance, inductance and impedance not seen when a constant current flows.

Inductance (L) is the property possessed by conductors in a circuit when alternating current flows. It controls the rate of change of current when a voltage is applied across the conductor.

$$L = \text{Potential/Rate of change of current}$$

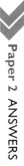

Reactance is the opposition to alternating current flow resulting from capacitance and inductance.

$$Reactance = Voltage/Current$$

Impedance (Z) is a measure of the sum of all the properties that resist the flow of an alternating current (inductance, reactance and capacitance).

$$Z = Voltage/Current$$

Further reading

Davey AJ, Diba A. *Ward's Anaesthetic Equipment*. 5th ed. Philadelphia: Elsevier Saunders; 2005. Chapter 2, p. 12–15.

41A: True
41B: True
41C: False
41D: True
41E: True

Catecholamines are substances whose chemical structure consists of a benzene ring with hydroxyl groups at positions 3 and 4 (*catechol-*) and an amine side chain (*-amine*). The naturally occurring catecholamines, dopamine, adrenaline and noradrenaline are synthesized from phenylalanine and tyrosine (phenylalanine is converted to tyrosine by phenylalanine hydroxylase) by a series of enzymes in a common pathway. Both naturally occurring and synthetic catecholamines (such as dopexamine and dobutamine) are used in the treatment of shock for their positive inotropic or vasopressor properties. They act via G-protein-coupled adrenoreceptors to alter intracellular cyclic AMP production. Their affinity for each of the receptor subtypes (α- and β-adrenoceptors and dopamine receptors) determines their effects, including positive inotropy, chronotropy, peripheral vasoconstriction or splanchnic vasodilatation.

Further reading

Stanchina ML, Levy MM. Vasoactive drug use in septic shock. *Semin Respir Crit Care Med*. 2004; 25(6): 673–681.

42A: False
42B: True
42C: False
42D: False
42E: True

The functional unit of the kidney is the nephron, which begins as the Bowman's capsule, collecting 125 ml·min^{-1} of glomerular filtrate formed by ultrafiltration of blood at the network of capillaries, which form the glomerulus. The glomerular filter is composed of the glomerular basement membrane, inter-digitating podocyte foot processes and capillary endothelial cells, and filters molecules by size, shape and charge. The glomerular basement membrane is mainly composed of negatively charged collagen, restricting passage of similarly negatively charged molecules and allowing only molecules less than 7 kDa molecular weight to be freely filtered. Molecules greater than 70 kDa are not filtered at all in health. Capillary endothelial cells contain fenestrations 60 nm in diameter, contributing to the filter by preventing passage of erythrocytes and platelets. The single nephron glomerular filtration rate is greatest in those found in the medulla.

Further reading

Lote CJ. *Principles of Renal Physiology*. 5th ed. New York: Springer; 2012.

43A: False
43B: True
43C: False
43D: True
43E: True

Magnesium is the fourth most abundant physiological cation (after sodium, potassium and calcium) and an important intracellular cation. Normal plasma concentrations of magnesium are 0.7–1.05 mmol·L^{-1}. This exists in both ionized and unionized forms, although only the ionized form is physiologically active. Approximately 50% of stored magnesium is found in soft tissue, with the remainder predominantly in bone, with less than 1% stored in erythrocytes. Magnesium is an essential cofactor in adenosine triphosphate (ATP)-dependent processes, chelating ATP to fully activate it. When present in high levels, magnesium directly inhibits both myocardial contractility and catecholamine receptors. In contrast, it enhances the positive inotropic effects of adrenaline. Magnesium causes vasodilatation directly as well as reducing the response of vascular smooth muscle to vasoconstrictors.

Further reading

Parikh M, Webb ST. Cations: potassium, calcium and magnesium. *Contin Educ Anaesth Crit Care Pain*. 2012; 12(4): 195–198.

Watson VF, Vaughan RS. Magnesium and the anaesthetist. *Contin Educ Anaesth Crit Care Pain*. 2001; 1(1): 16–20.

44A: True
44B: False
44C: True
44D: False
44E: True

Pulmonary blood flow (PBF) consists of flow from the right ventricle into the progressively branching pulmonary arteries, terminating at the pulmonary capillaries where gas exchange takes place with the alveolar gases. Both passive and active factors determine PBF and pulmonary vascular resistance (PVR) but passive factors predominate under normal physiological conditions. The PBF is equivalent to the cardiac output but is not uniform throughout the lung tissue. For example, blood flow in the upright patient is greater at the base than the apex of the lung; although blood flow in both upper and lower zones is increased during exercise due to recruitment and distension of capillaries. The lung can theoretically be divided into three 'zones' (described by West) where blood flow is determined by the relationship between arterial (P_A), alveolar (P_a) and venous pressures (P_v).

In the West zone 1, alveolar pressure exceeds both arterial and venous pressure and no blood flow is possible. In zone 2, the flow is determined by the difference between arterial and alveolar pressures, rather than in zone 3 where the usual arterio-venous pressure difference determines blood flow.

Hence:

West Zone 1: $P_A > P_a > P_v$
West Zone 2: $P_a > P_A > P_v$
West Zone 3: $P_a > P_v > P_A$

Further reading

West JB. Pulmonary blood flow and gas exchange. In *Respiratory Physiology: People and Ideas*. Oxford: Oxford University Press; 1996. p. 140–169.

West JB. Ventilation-perfusion inequality and overall gas exchange in computer models of the lung. *Respir Physiol*. 1969; 7: 88–110.

45A: False
45B: True
45C: False
45D: True
45E: False

The stretch reflex is the only monosynaptic reflex in the human body. This means that there is only one synapse between the afferent and efferent neurones of the reflex arc.

Intrafusal muscle fibres form sensory organs known as muscle spindles, which detect muscle fibre length.

When a whole muscle actively contracts muscle spindle relaxes and afferent axon firing stops.

When a muscle is passively stretched afferent axon firing increases (γ-motor fibres).

In order to maintain constant muscle fibre length, the following process occurs:

- Muscle stretch detected by muscle spindles
- Increased firing in muscle spindle afferent neurones
- These enter spinal cord via dorsal root
- Synapse in anterior horn with efferent fibres, muscle α-motor neurones
- These innervate extrafusal fibres, leading to contraction of the stretched muscle

Further reading

Cross M, Plunkett E. *Physics, Pharmacology and Physiology for Anaesthetists: Key Concepts for the FRCA*. Cambridge: Cambridge University Press; 2008.

Smith T, Pinnock C, Lin T. *Fundamentals of Anaesthesia*. 3rd ed. Cambridge: Cambridge University Press; 2009.

46A: False
46B: True
46C: False
46D: False
46E: True

Neurones are the main excitatory cell type within the nervous system. They are responsible for transmitting messages through the generation and propagation of action potentials.

- Action potential: the spontaneous depolarization of an excitable cell in response to a stimulus.

The electrical potential inside neurones at rest is negative with respect to the outside due to:

- Active transport of sodium ions out of the cell.
- Active transport of potassium ions into the cell.
- Passive diffusion of both potassium and sodium through the cell membrane but it is more permeable to potassium ions than sodium ions in the resting state. The membrane is impermeable to anions.

This is known as the resting membrane potential (–70 mV).

When a stimulus is received by the neurone, it responds by altering membrane ion permeability. If the stimulus is sufficient to achieve a membrane potential above threshold potential (–55 mV) an action potential will be generated.

Generation of an action potential:

- Above threshold potential, voltage-gated sodium channels open allowing rapid sodium influx into the cell. Membrane potential rises to +30 mV.
- Voltage-gated sodium channels close and potassium channels open. Potassium ions move out of the cell down their concentration gradient. Membrane potential drops again; this is repolarization.
- Membrane potential overshoots below resting membrane potential; this is hyperpolarization.
- Na^+/K^+-ATPase pump pumps sodium ions back out of the cell and potassium ions back into the cell to restore resting membrane potential.

Further reading

Cross M, Plunkett E. *Physics, Pharmacology and Physiology for Anaesthetists: Key Concepts for the FRCA*. Cambridge: Cambridge University Press; 2008.

Smith T, Pinnock C, Lin T. *Fundamentals of Anaesthesia*. 3rd ed. Cambridge: Cambridge University Press; 2009.

47A: True
47B: True
47C: False
47D: False
47E: False

The foetal circulation is adapted to receive oxygenated blood from the placenta via the umbilical vein, rather than from the pulmonary circulation as in the adult. This blood, which has an oxygen saturation of 80–90%, flows first towards the liver, where 50–60% bypasses the hepatic circulation into the ductus venosus. Blood from the ductus venosus enters the inferior vena cava (IVC) and then the right atrium (RA).

The IVC also receives deoxygenated blood with a saturation of 25–40% from the lower body and hepatic circulation. However, preferential streaming of oxygenated blood occurs and at the junction with the RA, a tissue flap known as the Eustachian valve directs the more oxygenated stream of blood towards the left atrium through an intracardiac shunt known as the foramen ovale.

This blood then enters the left ventricle and then is mostly delivered to the brain and coronary circulations via the ascending aorta, although some does join the descending aorta to the lower body.

Venous return from the superior vena cava and the deoxygenated stream of IVC blood enters the right ventricle from the RA and then proceeds to the pulmonary artery (PA). From the PA, 88% of blood bypasses the high resistance pulmonary circulation via another shunt known as the ductus arteriosus, leading to the descending aorta and supplying the lower body before returning to the placenta via the paired umbilical arteries.

Further reading

Murphy PJ. The fetal circulation. *Contin Educ Anaesth Crit Care Pain.* 2005; 5(4): 107–112.

48A: False
48B: True
48C: False
48D: True
48E: True

The brainstem consists of the midbrain, the medulla and the pons. It is the portion of the brain that, along with the cerebellum, sits below the tentorium. It is responsible for the control of autonomic function, consciousness as well as being the origin of numerous descending tracts and the site of a number of reflexes. It is also the location of the cranial nerves and their nuclei, and the respiratory control centres.

Brainstem function can be grossly tested in comatose patients by using brainstem reflexes.

The pupillary light reflex leads to pupillary constriction when the intensity of light to the pupil is significantly increased. This is mediated by the optic nerve (afferent) and the oculomotor nerve, and also assesses midbrain function.

The corneal reflex causes blinking when the cornea is stimulated by light touch. The afferent limb is composed of fibres of the trigeminal nerve, which supply sensation to the cornea; the efferent limb is the facial nerve that supplies the muscles of facial expression. It assesses brainstem function at the level of the pons.

The gag reflex tests the medulla. The afferent limb, the glossopharyngeal nerve, provides sensation to the posterior tongue, which is stimulated with a spatula, and the efferent limb produces a gag mediated by the vagus nerve, which provides motor supply to the pharynx and larynx.

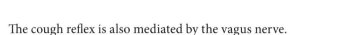

The cough reflex is also mediated by the vagus nerve.

The vestibulocochlear, or caloric reflex, results in eye movement and nystagmus when ice-cold water is introduced into the external auditory meatus. This is mediated by the vestibulocochlear nerve (afferent) and the third, fourth and sixth cranial nerves (which control eye movement) are the efferent limb.

Further reading

Academy of Medical Royal Colleges. *A Code of Practice for the Diagnosis and Confirmation of Death.* Academy of Medical Royal Colleges; 2008.

Gupta AK, Gelb AW. *Essentials of Neuroanaesthesia and Neurointensive Care.* Philadelphia: Saunders; 2008. Chapter 1.

49A: True
49B: True
49C: False
49D: False
49E: False

The peripheral chemoreceptors are located in the carotid bodies at the bifurcation of the common carotid artery and in the aortic bodies in the arch of the aorta. The chemoreceptors in the carotid bodies are the predominant chemoreceptors in humans. Central chemoreceptors are located near the ventral surface of the medulla. The central chemoreceptors are sensitive to changes in carbon dioxide tension but not oxygen. The peripheral chemoreceptors are also sensitive but only contribute less than 20% of the ventilatory response to a rise in carbon dioxide tension. The peripheral chemoreceptors are the source of response to hypoxia.

Baroreceptors are located in the aortic bodies and carotid sinuses. Stimulation of these by an increase in arterial blood pressure can cause reflex hypoventilation or apnoea. J-receptors are thought to be located in the alveolar walls (Juxtacapillary) and are supplied by the vagus nerve, which carries impulses to the brain.

Further reading

West JB. *Respiratory Physiology: The Essentials.* 9th ed. Philadelphia: Lippincott Williams & Wilkins; 2011.

50A: True
50B: False
50C: True
50D: True
50E: True

The principle effect of high altitude is an increase in the respiratory rate. This raises the alveolar oxygen partial pressure by reducing the partial pressure of carbon dioxide. This can be calculated using the alveolar gas equation. The stimulus for hyperventilation is hypoxia acting on the peripheral chemoreceptors. The resulting hyperventilation is limited by the decrease in arterial carbon dioxide and arterial alkalosis. Within one day at high altitude, the pH of the cerebrospinal fluid (CSF) returns to normal as bicarbonate moves out of the CSF. Over the next few days the serum pH returns to normal due to increased renal excretion of bicarbonate.

Acclimatization causes an increase in haemoglobin concentration through erythropoietin production from the kidney. This polycythemia serves to maintain the oxygen content of the blood in spite of reduced oxygen partial pressure and haemoglobin oxygen saturation. There is also an increase in the concentration of 2,3-diphosphoglycerate (2,3-DPG). The alveolar hypoxia causes pulmonary vasoconstriction, which increases the pulmonary arterial pressure and the strain on the right side of the heart. Changes also occur in the oxidative enzymes within cells and the capillary density of peripheral tissues increases.

Further reading

Brown J, Growcott M. Humans at altitude: physiology and pathophysiology. *Contin Educ Anaesth Crit Care Pain.* 2013; 13(1): 17–22.

Brown J, Growcott M. Humans at altitude: research and critical care. *Contin Educ Anaesth Crit Care Pain.* 2013; 13(1): 23–27.

51A: False
51B: True
51C: False
51D: False
51E: False

The sacrum is formed from the fusion of five rudimentary vertebrae. Its base articulates superiorly with the fifth lumbar vertebra and laterally with the ilia to form the sacroiliac joints. Inferiorly it articulates with the coccyx.

The sacral promontory lies on the anterior surface at the upper margin of the first sacral vertebrae. It bulges forward into the pelvic cavity. The sacral canal is formed from the sacral foramina and contains the cauda equina, filum terminale and meninges down to the lower border of the second sacral vertebra. The sacral hiatus, the site for a caudal block, is formed by the failure of fusion of the fifth and fourth laminae. The base of the sacrum is directed cephalad and it is connected with the inferior surface of the last lumbar vertebra.

Further reading

Snell RS. *Clinical Anatomy.* 7th ed. Philadelphia: Lippincott Williams & Wilkins; 2003.

52A: True
52B: False
52C: True
52D: False
52E: False

The lumbar plexus is formed by the anterior rami of the first four lumbar nerves. It is situated within the body of the psoas muscle and the nerves emerge from the lateral, medial and anterior surface of the muscle.

The branches are the:

- Iliohypogastric nerve (L1)
- Ilioinguinal nerve (L1)
- Lateral cutaneous nerve of the thigh (L2–3)
- Femoral nerve (L2,3,4)
- Genitofemoral nerve (L1–2)
- Obturator nerve (L2,3,4)

The lateral cutaneous nerve of the thigh as the name suggests is purely a sensory nerve. The genitofemoral nerve splits into a genital branch, which supplies the cremaster muscle and the femoral branch, which supplies sensation to skin on the thigh. The femoral nerve is the largest branch of the lumbar plexus.

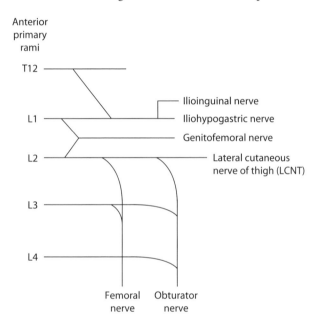

Further reading

Snell RS. *Clinical Anatomy*. 7th ed. Philadelphia: Lippincott Williams & Wilkins; 2003.

53A: False
53B: False
53C: False
53D: True
53E: True

The diaphragm is the most important muscle of respiration. Peripherally, it is muscular in nature and has a centrally placed tendon. It has three origins: a sternal part from the posterior part of the xiphoid process; a costal part from the inner surfaces of the lower six ribs; and a vertebral part. The right crus arises from the bodies of the first three lumbar vertebrae. In contrast the left crus arises from only the first two lumbar vertebrae. Laterally to the crura are the medial and lateral arcuate ligaments.

The diaphragm is innervated by the phrenic nerves that originate from the third to fifth cervical nerve roots ('C3,4,5 keeps the diaphragm alive'). The diaphragm has three openings. The most inferior is at the level of T12 and transmits the aorta, thoracic duct and azygos vein. Moving superiorly at the level of T10 the oesophagus passes through together with the right and left vagus nerves, oesophageal vessels and lymphatics from the lower third of the oesophagus. At T8 the vena cava passes together with branches of the right phrenic nerve.

Further reading

Snell RS. *Clinical Anatomy*. 7th ed. Philadelphia: Lippincott Williams & Wilkins; 2003.

54A: False
54B: True
54C: False
54D: True
54E: True

There are five roots to the brachial plexus, which are the anterior rami of the C5, 6, 7, 8 and T1 spinal nerve roots. The five roots give rise to three trunks: upper, middle and lower.

- The upper trunk is supplied by the C5 and 6
- The middle trunk is supplied by the C7
- The lower trunk is supplied by the C8 and T1

Each trunk divides to form two divisions: an anterior and a posterior one. Therefore, there are six divisions in total. The next section is composed of three cords. The cords are named according to their relation to the axillary artery.

- The posterior cord is formed from all three posterior divisions
- The lateral cord is formed from the anterior divisions of the upper and middle trunk
- The medial cord is the continuation of the anterior division of the lower trunk

The nerves of the brachial plexus are the branches and most arise from the cords. There are five terminal branches: musculocutaneous nerve, axillary nerve, radial nerve, median nerve and ulnar nerve. The lateral pectoral nerve arises from the lateral cord, whereas the long thoracic nerve (or the nerve of Bell) arises more proximally from the C5, 6, 7 nerve roots.

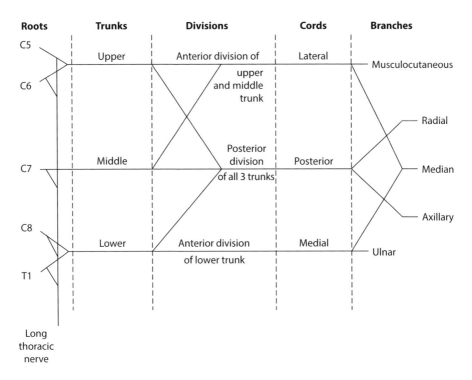

Roots	Trunks	Divisions	Cords	Branches

Long thoracic nerve

Further reading

Snell RS. *Clinical Anatomy*. 7th ed. Philadelphia: Lippincott Williams & Wilkins; 2003.

55A: False
55B: True
55C: True
55D: True
55E: True

The stress response is a combination of metabolic and hormonal changes that occur in response to surgery or trauma.

There are a number of mechanisms responsible for the stress response. Activation of the sympathetic nervous system renders the body prepared for a 'fight or flight' situation. The pituitary gland releases adrenocorticotrophic hormone (ACTH), growth hormone (GH), antidiuretic hormone (ADH) and prolactin. There is reduced insulin and increased glucagon release along with activation of the renin–angiotensin–aldosterone system.

The result is elevation of blood glucose level by hepatic gluconeogenesis and glycogenolysis in the presence of catecholamines, cortisol and low levels of insulin. Protein catabolism (in the presence of cortisol) causes muscle wasting, delayed wound healing and nitrogen loss in the urine. Lipolysis yields glycerol and free fatty acids, which are used for gluconeogenesis in the presence of catecholamines, cortisol and growth hormone. An increased circulating volume results from sodium and water retention in the presence of ADH and aldosterone.

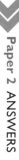

Further reading

Burton D, Nicholson G, Hall G. Endocrine and metabolic response to surgery. *Contin Educ Anaesth Crit Care Pain.* 2004; 4(5): 144–147.

56A: False
56B: True
56C: True
56D: True
56E: False

The resting membrane potential (RMP) is the potential difference present across the cell membrane when no stimulation is occurring. It is caused by the differing concentrations of ions that are present in and out of the cell. The intracellular environment is 70–80 mV more negative than the extracellular environment, largely due to the presence of anionic proteins. The Gibbs–Donnan effect describes the existence of a chemical gradient, along which ions move to equilibrate. Full chemical equilibrium is prevented from occurring, however, as the existence of an opposing electrical potential prevents further movement of ions. The ions therefore move until an electrochemical equilibrium is achieved.

Nernst calculated the potential difference that an ion would produce if the membrane were freely permeable to that ion. The resting membrane potential is thus similar to the Nernst potential for potassium as the membrane is freely permeable to potassium. The Na^+/K^+ pump moves 3 Na^+ ions out of the cell and 2 K^+ ions into the cell, hence increases the RMP by making the intracellular environment more negative.

Saltatory (from the Latin *saltare*, 'to leap') conduction occurs along myelinated nerve fibres between nodes of Ranvier and results in more rapid propagation of the action potential.

Further reading

Power I, Kam P. *Principles of Physiology for the Anaesthetist.* 2nd ed. London: Hodder Arnold; 2008.

Smith T, Pinnock C, Lin T. *Fundamentals of Anaesthesia.* 3rd ed. Cambridge: Cambridge University Press; 2009. p. 253–258.

57A: False
57B: True
57C: True
57D: True
57E: True

Fatty acid metabolism occurs predominantly in the mitochondrial matrix by a process known as beta oxidation. Free fatty acids in the cytoplasm are activated by esterification with acetyl-CoA. The activated fatty acid is loaded onto a carrier protein on the outer membrane of the mitochondrion and transported across the membrane into the mitochondrial matrix, where it combines with acetyl-CoA once again. This transmembrane carrier process is known as the carnitine shuttle. Inside the mitochondrion, two carbon fragments are broken from the fatty acid in repeated steps, producing acetyl-CoA, which enters the citric acid cycle. It can be seen that fatty acid metabolism yields more acetyl-CoA than glucose metabolism, hence has a greater energy yield.

Further reading

Smith T, Pinnock C, Lin T. *Fundamentals of Anaesthesia*. 3rd ed. Cambridge: Cambridge University Press; 2009. p. 253–258.

58A: False
58B: True
58C: False
58D: True
58E: True

The autonomic nervous system (ANS) is a collection of nerves and ganglia that are responsible for the maintenance of homeostasis and coordination of the stress response. The ANS controls visceral organs, smooth muscle and secretory glands and is involuntary, hence 'autonomic'.

Parasympathetic nerve fibres are cranio-sacral in origin. Parasympathetic ganglia are located near effector sites, with short postganglionic fibres, which release acetylcholine as a neurotransmitter. Cranial nerves with parasympathetic fibres are the oculomotor, facial, glossopharyngeal and vagus nerves (III, VII, IX, X).

- Oculomotor (III): from the oculomotor nucleus, parasympathetic fibres pass through the orbit to the ciliary ganglion, where postganglionic fibres pass to the ciliary muscle and constrict the pupil.
- Facial (VII): from the superior salivary nucleus of the facial nerve, fibres form chorda tympani to the lingual nerve and the submaxillary ganglion. Postganglionic fibres then pass to the submandibular and sublingual salivary glands.
- Glossopharyngeal (IX): parasympathetic fibres from the salivary nucleus of the glossopharyngeal nerve innervate the parotid gland.
- Vagus (X): preganglionic fibres from the dorsal nucleus of the vagus nerve in the medulla terminate in ganglia and plexus of visceral organs.
  - Cardiovascular innervation of the SA node, atria and AV node slows the heart rate and reduces atrial contraction
  - Respiratory innervation causes bronchoconstriction
  - Gastric innervation causes increased motility and relaxation of the pyloric sphincter

Further reading

Power I, Kam P. *Principles of Physiology for the Anaesthetist*. 2nd ed. London: Hodder Arnold; 2008.

Smith T, Pinnock C, Lin T. *Fundamentals of Anaesthesia*. 3rd ed. Cambridge: Cambridge University Press; 2009. p. 253–258.

59A: False
59B: True
59C: True
59D: True
59E: False

Agglutinogens (antigens) exist on the surface of red blood cells. There are over 400 types of antigens; however, they differ in their ability to cause immune reactions. ABO and rhesus groups account for the majority of clinically significant transfusion incompatibility reactions.

A, B and O genes are responsible for the production of enzymes that catalyze the addition of specific carbohydrate groups to the core red cell antigen (the H antigen). This process results in the production of 'A' and 'B' red cell antigens, which are expressed on the surface of the red cell and determine the ABO blood group. Patients who lack either the A or B antigen produce natural antibodies to these antigens.

Group	Antigen on RBC	Antibody in Serum	Donate Blood to	Receive Blood from
AB	A, B	Nil	AB	O, A, B, AB
A	A	Anti B	A, AB	A, O
B	B	Anti A	B, AB	O, B
O	None	Anti A, Anti B	A, B, AB, O	O

As the table demonstrates, patients who have blood type O are considered universal donors. Patients who have blood type AB are therefore known as universal receivers.

Haemolytic transfusion reactions are immune-mediated reactions that occur in cases of ABO incompatibility. Immediate intravascular haemolysis occurs and causes the clinical features of urticarial rash and flushing, back pain, chest pain, breathlessness and rigors. Cardiovascular collapse may ensue with multi-organ failure. In the United Kingdom, haemolytic transfusion reactions are rare and are usually due to clerical errors.

Regarding the second stem, in the UK the most prevalent blood types in descending order are O, A, B, AB. Therefore, someone with a B antigen is more likely to react to group A blood than not.

Further reading

Maxwell MJ, Wilson MJA. Complications of blood transfusion. *Contin Educ Anaesth Crit Care Pain.* 2006; 6(6): 225–229.

Power I, Kam P. *Principles of Physiology for the Anaesthetist.* 2nd ed. London: Hodder Arnold; 2008.

60A: True
60B: False
60C: True
60D: True
60E: True

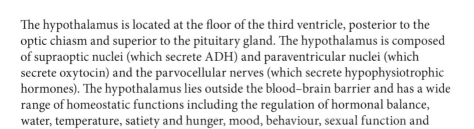

The hypothalamus is located at the floor of the third ventricle, posterior to the optic chiasm and superior to the pituitary gland. The hypothalamus is composed of supraoptic nuclei (which secrete ADH) and paraventricular nuclei (which secrete oxytocin) and the parvocellular nerves (which secrete hypophysiotrophic hormones). The hypothalamus lies outside the blood–brain barrier and has a wide range of homeostatic functions including the regulation of hormonal balance, water, temperature, satiety and hunger, mood, behaviour, sexual function and autonomic functions.

Hypophysiotrophic hormones are secreted by the hypothalamus into the portal circulation to the anterior pituitary, where they regulate the synthesis and release of anterior pituitary hormones. The hypophysiotrophic hormones are: gonadotrophin releasing hormone, growth hormone releasing hormone, somatostation, thyroid releasing hormone, dopamine, corticotrophin releasing hormone and prolactin releasing hormone.

ADH and oxytocin are synthesized by the hypothalamus and packaged into granules, which pass along neuronal axons to be stored in the posterior pituitary.

Further reading

Menon R, Renon PG. Anaesthesia and pituitary disease. *Contin Educ Anaesth Crit Care Pain*. 2011; 11(4): 133–137.

Power I, Kam P. *Principles of Physiology for the Anaesthetist*. 2nd ed. London: Hodder Arnold; 2008.

1. **Side effects of etomidate include:**
   A. Epileptiform activity on the EEG in up to 20% of patients
   B. Postoperative nausea and vomiting
   C. Increased intracranial pressure
   D. Inhibition of 11β-hydroxylase
   E. Pain on injection

2. **The following block reuptake of noradrenaline:**
   A. Nortryptilline
   B. Phenelzine
   C. Clonidine
   D. Venlafaxine
   E. Tranylcypromine

3. **The following are effects of anticholinesterase drugs:**
   A. Depolarizing neuromuscular blockade
   B. Bradycardia
   C. Elevated intraocular pressure
   D. Bronchospasm
   E. Constipation

4. **Partial agonists:**
   A. Have a lower affinity for the receptor than the agonist
   B. Can produce a maximal response at the receptor if given in large enough doses
   C. Are antagonists when combined with an agonist
   D. Have a lower efficacy than full agonists
   E. Have a lower potency than full agonists

5. **Cannabinoids:**
   A. Are derived from cannabis
   B. Are hydrophilic compounds
   C. Exert their effect by non-specific membrane interactions
   D. Are derived from arachidonic acid
   E. Their prescription is illegal in the United Kingdom

6. The following drug combinations can give rise to serotonin syndrome:
A. Sertraline and isocarboxazid
B. Linezolid and paroxetine
C. Moclobemide and pethidine
D. Amitriptyline and tranylcypromine
E. Phenelzine and phenylephrine

7. Dantrolene:
A. Limits the accumulation of calcium ions in skeletal muscle cells
B. Is prepared with mannitol to improve solubility
C. When used to treat malignant hyperthermia, the initial dose is 10 mg·kg^{-1}
D. Is a hydantoin derivative
E. Is used prophylactically in the majority of individuals susceptible to malignant hyperthermia who are undergoing anaesthesia

8. Adrenaline is used:
A. In an intravenous dose of 1 mg in the treatment of asystole in adults
B. In an intramuscular dose of 500 micrograms in the treatment of anaphylaxis
C. In a concentration of 1:200 000 in combination with local anaesthetic solutions
D. As a 10% topical solution in the treatment of glaucoma
E. In an intravenous dose of 50 micrograms (0.5 mL of 1:100 000 solution) in the treatment of anaphylaxis

9. The following drugs contain a benzyl group:
A. Remifentanil
B. Neostigmine
C. Lignocaine
D. Suxamethonium
E. Aspirin

10. Hepatoxicity is commonly caused by the following chemotherapy agents:
A. Cisplatin
B. Vincristine
C. Vinblastine
D. Bleomycin
E. 5-flurouracil

11. The following drugs are naturally occurring catecholamines:
A. Dopamine
B. Phenylephrine
C. Adrenaline
D. Isoprenaline
E. Ephedrine

12. When using target controlled infusions:
A. The Marsh model uses patient age in its calculation
B. The Schneider model calculates lean body mass
C. The elderly have a lower central volume of distribution
D. The algorithms use three superimposed infusions
E. The Marsh and Schneider models calculate the same value for volume of the central compartment

13. The following antiemetics are dopamine antagonists:
A. Cyclizine
B. Domperidone
C. Ondansetron
D. Metoclopramide
E. Prochlorperazine

14. Drugs that induce hepatic cytochrome P450 include:
A. Grapefruit juice
B. Isoniazid
C. Phenytoin
D. Halothane
E. Metronidazole

15. The following drugs are selective phosphodiesterase III inhibitors:
A. Isoprenaline
B. Enoximone
C. Milrinone
D. Aminophylline
E. Isoprenaline

16. Side effects of suxamethonium include:
A. Hyperkalaemia
B. Bradycardia
C. Seizures
D. Myalgia
E. Tachycardia

17. The following drugs prolong QT interval:
A. Digoxin
B. Suxamethonium
C. Citalopram
D. Amiodarone
E. Bendroflumethiazide

18. The following drugs are Vaughan–Williams class III anti-arrhythmics:
A. Sotalol
B. Metoprolol
C. Digoxin
D. Disopyramide
E. Amiodarone

19. Metabolism of the following drugs is affected by genetic polymorphisms:
   A. Isoniazid
   B. Suxamethonium
   C. Codeine
   D. Remifentanil
   E. Hydralazine

20. The following antimicrobials act on the 30S ribosomal subunit:
   A. Clindamycin
   B. Vancomycin
   C. Gentamicin
   D. Erythromycin
   E. Metronidazole

21. Regarding temperature measurement:
   A. The linear relationship between the resistance of a conductor and its temperature is known as the Seebeck effect
   B. A Wheatstone bridge is commonly used in conjunction with a thermistor
   C. The Stewart–Hamilton law refers to the concept of a black body, where an ideal object emits an equal amount of infrared energy as that given to it
   D. Semi-conductors exhibit a linear decline in resistance with increasing temperature
   E. The resistance thermometer is more sensitive than the thermistor

22. The heat and moisture exchange device:
   A. May be obstructed by respiratory secretions
   B. Demonstrates improved performance with low fresh gas flows
   C. Warms inspired gases to greater than 34°C
   D. Demonstrates improved performance by increasing the volume of the hygrophobic medium
   E. Delivers a relative humidity of 30 g·m^{-3} of water vapour at 30°C

23. Components of the Severinghaus CO_2 electrode are:
   A. A reference silver/silver chloride electrode
   B. Potassium hydroxide solution
   C. Hydrogen-sensitive glass
   D. Hydrochloric acid buffer
   E. A reference mercury/mercury chloride electrode

24. A 50-Hz alternating current passing through a hand will predominantly cause:
   A. Tingling sensation at 75 mA
   B. Severe pain at 15 mA
   C. Ventricular fibrillation at 50 mA
   D. Respiratory arrest at 15 mA
   E. Atrial fibrillation at 75 mA

25. The following definitions regarding decontamination are correct:
  A. Cleaning is the physical removal of foreign material
  B. Sterilization destroys all forms of bacterial life but not viruses
  C. Disinfection eliminates all pathogenic organisms except bacterial spores
  D. Examples of disinfectants include ethylene oxide and gutaraldehyde
  E. For prevention of prion disease transmission, sterilization is required

26. Regarding ventilators:
  A. Mechanical thumbs are not suitable for the paediatric population
  B. The Manley MP3 ventilator is an example of a minute volume divider
  C. The Penlon Nuffield series ventilators are examples of mechanical thumbs
  D. Bag squeezers are rarely used during anaesthesia but more commonly in intensive care ventilation
  E. Only intermittent blowers require a pressurized source of gas

27. The following statements are correct:
  A. Mainstream capnography incorporates a sapphire windowed chamber, which is heated to 61°C
  B. Sidestream capnography draws sample gas at a flow rate of approximately 150–200 ml·min^{-1}
  C. The external diameter of the sample tubing in sidestream capnography is 1–2 mm
  D. Sidestream capnography has a lag time of 2.5–3 seconds, depending on the length of tubing used
  E. Mainstream infrared spectrometers are currently only used for carbon dioxide

28. The following statements regarding intravenous equipment are correct:
  A. Manually controlled adult giving sets produce 20 drops of clear fluid per millilitre
  B. All blood products should be administered through a giving set with a filter of 150 micrometre mesh
  C. Paediatric giving sets produce 30 drops of clear fluid per millilitre
  D. Blood giving sets are of narrower diameter to prevent red cell haemolysis
  E. The addition of 0.2 micrometre filters to paediatric giving sets reduces the incidence of thrombophlebitis

29. Volumetric pumps:
  A. Are most suitable for infusions requiring a precise flow rate
  B. Are accurate to within 2%
  C. Are used for infusions at flow rates greater than 5 ml·hr^{-1}
  D. Should not be positioned above the patient
  E. Have an alarm system that detects air in the infusion line

30. A capacitor:
  A. Has high resistance to DC signals
  B. Has high reactance to AC signals
  C. Has a greater capacitance if large capacitor plates are used
  D. Has a greater capacitance if the plates are close together
  E. Has high impedance to low-frequency signals

31. **The following statements regarding electricity are correct:**
    A. The coulomb is the unit of electrical current
    B. One volt is the potential difference between two points on a conducting wire carrying 1 ampere of current, between which 1 watt of power is dissipated
    C. One volt is equal to 10 joules per coulomb
    D. One ampere contains 6.24×10^{18} electrons
    E. A thick wire has a lower resistance than a thin wire

32. **Which of the following are recommended by the Association of Anaesthetists of Great Britain and Ireland (AAGBI) as essential monitoring components during anaesthesia:**
    A. Oxygen analyzer with an audible alarm
    B. Monitoring of ambient anaesthetic concentrations
    C. Carbon dioxide analyzer
    D. Anaesthetic vapour analyzer
    E. Carbon dioxide alarm

33. **Non-invasive blood pressure measurement using a cuff system:**
    A. Is entirely safe
    B. Is always comfortable for the patient
    C. Should be measured on the uppermost limb when in the lateral position
    D. Is inaccurate in the presence of arrhythmias
    E. Is accurate over a wide range of blood pressures

34. **The following definitions are correct:**
    A. True positive: the patient has the disease and the test is positive
    B. True negative: the patient has the disease but the test is negative
    C. Sensitivity: the ability of a test to correctly identify those patients with the disease
    D. Specificity: the sum of the true negatives and false positives divided by the true negatives
    E. Positive predictive value: how likely is it that this patient has the disease given the test is positive

35. **The following situations pose a fire risk:**
    A. Ether in air heated to 200°C
    B. Halothane in oxygen
    C. Betadine and diathermy
    D. Ethyl chloride in nitrous oxide
    E. Using Vaseline® as lubricant on a reducing valve

36. **When measuring lung volumes:**
    A. The helium dilution method measures the total volume of gas in the lung
    B. A spirometer measures all lung volumes and capacities except residual volume
    C. In the helium dilution technique the patient is connected to the spirometer after a maximal expiration
    D. Helium is used due to its low solubility in blood
    E. The body plethysmograph uses the principle of Boyle's law

37. **The following pairings are incorrect:**
    A. Normally distributed data from two groups: Student's t-test
    B. Non-normally distributed data from two groups: Kruskal-Wallis test
    C. Normally distributed data from more than two groups: ANOVA
    D. Non-normally distributed data from more than two groups: Mann-Whitney U-test
    E. Qualitative data: Chi-squared test

38. **The following statements about damping and resonance are correct:**
    A. In an arterial pressure monitoring system the natural frequency of the system should be above 400 Hz
    B. In an underdamped system no overshooting occurs
    C. A critically damped system has a damping factor of 1.0
    D. An overdamped system has a damping factor of <0.7
    E. Damping can be caused by excessively stiff tubing in the system

39. **The Bain breathing system:**
    A. Is more efficient with positive pressure ventilation than with the spontaneously breathing patient
    B. Requires fresh gas flows 2–3 times higher than alveolar ventilation to prevent rebreathing during spontaneous ventilation
    C. Requires fresh gas flows of 70–100 ml·kg^{-1}·min^{-1} to prevent rebreathing in a positively pressure ventilated patient
    D. If the inner tube is disconnected at the machine end, the dead space is reduced
    E. The volume of the expiratory limb is approximately 700 ml

40. **The following definitions regarding mathematical relationships are correct:**
    A. A linear relationship can be expressed as $y = mx + c$, where m is the point of crossing the x axis
    B. In an exponential function, the rate of change of a variable at any point in time is proportional to the value of the variable at that time
    C. Boyle's law is an example of a hyperbolic function
    D. $y = kx^2$ describes a hyperbolic relationship
    E. $\log(xy) = \log(x) \times \log(y)$

41. **Chloride:**
    A. Is the most abundant intracellular anion
    B. Is important in gastric acid production
    C. Is reabsorbed in the proximal convoluted tubule
    D. Contributes to strong ion difference
    E. Moves into erythrocytes as bicarbonate diffuses out

42. **Renal blood flow:**
    A. To the inner medulla is 50 ml·100g^{-1}·min^{-1}
    B. Is 20–25% of cardiac output at rest
    C. Exhibits autoregulation between mean arterial pressures of 50–150 mmHg
    D. Is approximately 600 ml·min^{-1}
    E. Can be determined from clearance of para-aminohippuric acid (PAH)

43. Functional residual capacity is reduced by:
 A. Pregnancy
 B. Standing up
 C. Increasing age
 D. Lung fibrosis
 E. Asthma

44. Closing volume (CV):
 A. Is the volume of air remaining in the lung after forced expiration
 B. Can be measured by nitrogen washout
 C. Is greater than functional residual capacity in neonates
 D. Is less than functional residual capacity in pregnant women
 E. Is increased by general anaesthesia

45. Risk factors for postoperative nausea and vomiting (PONV) include:
 A. Male gender
 B. Non-smoker
 C. Strabismus surgery
 D. Inadequate analgesia
 E. Obesity

46. Regarding iron:
 A. 50% of ingested iron is absorbed
 B. Haem and non-haem iron is absorbed by pinocytosis
 C. Free iron is stored as ferritin by binding to apoferritin
 D. 70% of body iron is in haemoglobin
 E. Absorption of iron depends on total body stores

47. For carbon dioxide transport in the blood:
 A. In arterial blood 5% is dissolved
 B. It is 40 times more soluble than oxygen
 C. The Hamburger effect involves chloride exchange for bicarbonate in red blood cells
 D. In venous blood 90% is transported as carbonic acid
 E. It binds predominantly to albumin to form carbamino compounds

48. Regarding the baroreceptor reflex:
 A. Baroreceptors are found in the atria and ventricles
 B. Carotid sinus baroreceptors transmit impulses via the vagus nerve
 C. Increased blood pressure stimulates the medullary vasomotor centre
 D. Aortic baroreceptor stimulation causes tachycardia
 E. Baroreceptors can respond to changes in heart rate

49. Regarding haemoglobin defects:
 A. They are the most common of all genetic disorders
 B. There are four α-globin genes
 C. β-Thalassaemia is diagnosed at birth
 D. The P50 for HbS is higher than for HbA
 E. In sickle cell disease there is a mutation resulting in a single substitution of an amino acid in the globin molecule

50. The following statements regarding gastric hormones are correct:
   A. Gastrin is secreted by G cells in the duodenum
   B. Somatostatin is released by S cells in the stomach
   C. Cholecystokinin is released by I cells in the small intestine
   D. Gastrin secretion is stimulated by drinking wine and coffee
   E. Secretin secretion is stimulated by increased acidity in the stomach

51. For pain pathways:
   A. The cell bodies of peripheral nociceptors are located in the dorsal root ganglia in the spinal cord
   B. Rexed laminae VII-IX make up the dorsal horn of the spinal cord
   C. Nociceptive information is transmitted mainly by the spinothalamic tract
   D. The antero-lateral funiculus is composed of the lateral spinothalamic tract, spinoreticular tract and spinomesencephalic tract
   E. The spinothalamic tract decussates at the level of the medulla

52. The following statements about the larynx are correct:
   A. It is made up of eight individual cartilages
   B. All the intrinsic muscles are innervated by the recurrent laryngeal nerve
   C. The vestibular folds are innervated by the internal laryngeal nerve
   D. A palsy of the external laryngeal nerve leads to difficulty in relaxing the vocal cords
   E. The posterior cricoarytenoid muscles abduct the vocal cords

53. The following pairings for dermatomes are correct:
   A. Occiput of the head: C1
   B. Axilla: T1
   C. Middle finger: C7
   D. Great toe: L5
   E. Anal margin: S5

54. For the anatomy of the back:
   A. The ligamentum flavum connects adjacent vertebral spines
   B. The interspinous ligaments connect adjacent vertebral laminae
   C. In adults the spinal cord usually terminates at the lower border of the first lumbar vertebrae
   D. As the anterior and posterior rami pass through the intervertebral foramina they unite to form the spinal nerves
   E. The conus medullaris is composed of the roots of the lumbar and sacral nerves below the termination of the cord

55. During starvation:
   A. Glycogen stores are exhausted after 7 days
   B. Protein catabolism occurs late
   C. Glucose requirements fall
   D. Gluconeogenesis is stimulated by low glucagon levels
   E. β-hydroxybutyrate can be used as a fuel source by the brain

56. Activation of the following receptors causes nausea:
A. Mechanoreceptors in the stomach, supplied by the glossopharyngeal nerve
B. Dopaminergic (D1) receptors in the chemoreceptor trigger zone
C. Chemoreceptors in the gut supplied by the vagus nerve
D. Opioid (μ) receptors in the chemoreceptor trigger zone
E. Histaminic (H1) receptors in the chemoreceptor trigger zone

57. Compared with plasma, cerebrospinal fluid (CSF) contains:
A. More potassium
B. Less protein
C. More sodium
D. More bicarbonate
E. A lower partial pressure of carbon dioxide

58. Sources of ammonia include:
A. Aspartate
B. Glutamine
C. Urea
D. Deoxyribonucleic acid
E. Beta-hydroxybutyrate

59. The following are exocrine secretions of the pancreas:
A. Insulin
B. Trypsinogen
C. Glucagon
D. Bicarbonate
E. Amylase

60. Type 1 skeletal muscle fibres:
A. Are slow oxidative fibres
B. Have few mitochondria
C. Are the predominant fibre type in oculomotor muscles
D. Have a high oxidative capacity
E. Depend largely on glycolysis for fuel metabolism

1A: True
1B: True
1C: False
1D: True
1E: True

Etomidate is a carboxylated imidazole derivative that is used for the induction of general anaesthesia and as a treatment to reduce steroidogenesis prior to surgery for Cushing syndrome. Etomidate has a number of favourable properties (rapid onset, cardiovascular stability on induction); however, it is not widely used due to its side-effect profile.

Pharmacodynamic effects of etomidate are:

- Cardiovascular: maintenance of sympathetic tone with slight reduction in mean arterial pressure, tachycardia in high doses
- Respiratory: dose-related respiratory depression, transient apnoea, hiccoughs and coughing, no inhibition of airway reflexes in response to laryngoscopy
- Central nervous system: rapid induction of general anaesthesia, involuntary muscle movements, tremor, hypertonus and a reduction in intracranial pressure, intraocular pressure, cerebral blood flow and cerebral metabolic rate, epileptiform activity on the EEG
- Gastrointestinal: nausea and vomiting
- Metabolic/endocrine: inhibition of steroid synthesis in the adrenal cortex (reversible inhibition of 11 β-hydroxylase and 17 α-hydroxylase causing a reduction in cortisol and aldosterone synthesis for at least 24 hours following a single dose); etomidate infusion in septic patients is associated with a high incidence of mortality due to steroid inhibition
- Haematological: antiplatelet effects

Other side effects of etomidate are pain on injection, venous thrombosis (due to preparation with ethylene glycol) and myoclonus.

Further reading

Forman SA. Clinical and molecular pharmacology of etomidate. *Anaesthesiology.* 2011; 114(3): 695–707.

2A: True
2B: False
2C: False
2D: True
2E: False

The monoamine hypothesis of depression proposes that depletion of neurotransmitters (noradrenaline, serotonin) in certain central pathways leads to depression and psychosis. Pharmacological treatment of depression acts by increasing levels of these neurotransmitters within the central nervous system (CNS).

Tricyclic antidepressants (TCAs; e.g. amitryptilline, dosulepin, nortryptilline, imipramine), act by blocking presynaptic uptake of noradrenaline and serotonin, resulting in increased concentration of these neurotransmitters in the synapse. These agents are used in the treatment of depression, acute and chronic pain and nocturnal enuresis. TCAs also block histamine, muscarinic and α-adrenoceptors. Side effects of TCAs are sedation, reduced seizure threshold in epileptics, anticholinergic side effects and postural hypotension (particularly in the elderly due to α-adrenoceptor blockade). These agents potentiate indirect acting sympathomimetic agents, interact with tramadol to cause serotonin syndrome and cause cholinergic symptoms if withdrawn abruptly.

Venlafaxine is a selective serotonin and noradrenaline reuptake inhibitor (SNRI), which is used as a second line antidepressant. Venlafaxine has few side effects but may also precipitate serotonin syndrome.

Monoamine oxidase inhibitors (MAOIs) are less frequently used due to an unfavourable side effect profile. MAOIs may be selective for the MAO type A enzyme (e.g. meclobemide) or non-selective (e.g. phenelzine, tranylcypromine, isocarboxazid). MAOIs potentiate the action of indirect sympathomimetics and may result in a hypertensive crisis.

Further reading

Peck T, Wong A, Norman E. Anaesthetic implications of psychoactive drugs. *Contin Educ Anaesth Crit Care Pain*. 2010; 10(6): 177–181.

3A: True
3B: True
3C: False
3D: True
3E: False

Anticholinesterase drugs act by inhibiting the breakdown of acetylcholine (ACh) in the neuronal synapse, prolonging its existence at the cholinergic receptors. The clinical effects seen are equivalent to excessive parasympathetic stimulation.

- Neuromuscular junction
  - Competitive inhibition of neuromuscular blocking drugs
  - Depolarizing block in overdose due to excess ACh present in synapse, repeatedly depolarizing the motor endplate
  - Fasciculation due to excess ACh causing repeated depolarization of motor endplate

- Cardiovascular
  - Bradycardia
- Respiratory
  - Increased secretions
  - Bronchospasm
- Gastrointestinal
  - Increased motility (vomiting, diarrhoea)
  - Incontinence
- Ocular
  - Miosis
  - Reduced intraocular pressure due to facilitation of the outflow of aqueous humour

Further reading

Priya Nair V, Hunter JM. Anticholinesterases and anticholinergic drugs. *Contin Educ Anaesth Crit Care Pain.* 2004; 4(5): 164–168.

4A: False
4B: False
4C: True
4D: True
4E: False

The two properties of a drug that determine its interaction with a receptor are:

1. The affinity of the drug (how well it binds to the receptor)
2. The intrinsic activity or efficacy of the drug (the magnitude of effect once the drug has bound, i.e. 0 to 1; in the case of inverse agonists the intrinsic activity would be –1)

From this we can define drugs as agonists or antagonists.

- Agonist: drug with significant receptor affinity and full intrinsic activity (IA = 1). Binding of the drug produces the maximal effect that receptor is capable of producing, for example, morphine at the μ-opioid receptor.
- Antagonist: drug with significant receptor affinity but no intrinsic activity (IA – 0), for example, ketamine at the NMDA receptor.
- Partial agonist: drug with significant receptor affinity and fractional intrinsic activity (IA <1), for example, buprenorphine at the μ-opioid receptor.

Potency is a measure of the dose or plasma drug concentration at which a response occurs. A potent drug causes a response at a low plasma drug concentration (or dose).

Further reading

Lambert DG. Drugs and receptors. *Contin Educ Anaesth Crit Care Pain.* 2004; 4(6): 181–184.

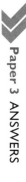
5A: True
5B: False
5C: False
5D: True
5E: False

Cannabinoids (CBs) are chemical compounds derived from the cannabis plant, *Cannabis sativa*. They are low molecular weight lipophilic compounds of approximately 300 Da in weight. Initial studies showed a direct correlation of psychoactivity with disruption of artificial lipid membranes. It was thought they functioned via non-specific membrane interactions. It has since been shown that cannabinoids exert their effect through G-protein coupled receptors (CBRs). There are around 60 phytocannabinoids obtained from the cannabis plant, which are a mix of agonists, partial agonists and antagonists at the CBRs. The discovery of CBRs led to the identification of endogenous cannabinoid ligands, which are derived from arachidonic acid.

Tincture of cannabis was available for prescription in the United Kingdom until 1971. Currently, CBs are licensed as antiemetics in chemotherapy and can be prescribed on a named basis for neuropathic pain.

Further reading

Hosking RD, Zajicek JP. Therapeutic potential of cannabis in pain medicine. *Br J Anaesth.* 2008; 101(1): 59–68.

6A: True
6B: True
6C: True
6D: False
6E: False

Serotonin toxicity is described as a triad of neuro-excitatory features:

- Neuromuscular hyperactivity: tremor, clonus, myoclonus, hyper-reflexia and pyramidal rigidity
- Autonomic hyperactivity: agitation, fever, tachycardia and tachypnoea
- Altered mental state: agitation, excitement and confusion

Serotonin toxicity is usually rapid and occurs due to drug combinations and begins when the second drug reaches effective plasma levels. It is reliably diagnosed if, in the presence of a serotonergic agent, spontaneous clonus is present. This can be confused with neuroleptic malignant syndrome.

The drug combinations that are likely to cause serotonin syndrome are monoamine oxidase inhibitors (MAOIs) with serotonin reuptake inhibitors. Serotonin releasers when combined with MAOIs will have the same effect too.

Serotonin Re-Uptake Inhibitors	Serotonin Releasers	Monoamine Oxidase Inhibitors
Paroxetine, sertraline	MDMA	Tranylcypromine
Venlafaxine		Phenelzine
Clomipramine, imipramine (not other TCAs)		Isocarboxazid
Tramadol, pethidine, fentanyl, methadone		Moclobemide
Chlorpheniramine		Linezolid

Further reading

Gillman PK. Monoamine oxidase inhibitors, opioid analgesics and serotonin toxicity. *Br J Anaesth*. 2005; 95(4): 434–441.

7A: True
7B: True
7C: False
7D: True
7E: False

Dantrolene is a phenyl hydantoin derivative, which is used in the management of malignant hyperthermia (MH) and in the prevention and treatment of muscle spasm in patients with spinal cord injury, tetanus and neuroleptic malignant syndrome. Dantrolene causes muscle relaxation by inhibition of the ryanodine receptor on the sarcoplasmic reticulum in skeletal muscle cells to reduce the accumulation of intracellular calcium ions. Dantrolene is prepared in an ampoule as a lyophilized orange powder containing 20 mg dantrolene sodium, 3 g mannitol (to increase solubility) and sodium bicarbonate. Each vial is reconstituted with 60 mL water, which can be labour intensive in an emergency. The usual initial dose in the management of malignant hyperthermia is a 2.5 mg·kg^{-1} bolus, followed by additional 1 mg·kg^{-1} boluses as required up to a maximum of 10 mg·kg^{-1}. Dantrolene is not routinely used in the prophylaxis of MH in susceptible individuals due to the occurrence of side effects such as sedation, muscle weakness (especially respiratory), gastrointestinal upset and hepatic dysfunction.

Further reading

AAGBI Safety Guideline. Malignant hyperthermia crisis. 2011. [Online] Available from: http://www.aagbi.org/sites/default/files/mh_guideline_for_website.pdf.

Halsall PJ, Hopkins PM. Malignant hyperthermia. *Contin Educ Anaesth Crit Care Pain*. 2003; 3(1): 5–9.

8A: True
8B: True
8C: True
8D: False
8E: False

Synthetic adrenaline is used at different doses to treat a number of conditions.

One ampoule of 1:1000 adrenaline contains 1 mg adrenaline (1000 micrograms·mL^{-1}). If 1 mL of 1:1000 adrenaline is diluted into 10 mL, a solution of 1:10 000 adrenaline is produced, with 1 mg in 10 mL (100 micrograms·mL^{-1}).

Adrenaline is used in the treatment of anaphylaxis at a bolus dose of 500 micrograms intramuscular injection (0.5 mL of 1:1000 concentration solution), or 50 micrograms intravenous injection (0.5 mL of 1:10 000 concentration solution or 5 mL of 1:100 000 solution, which is more practical to handle).

It is used in the treatment of adult cardiac arrest at a bolus dose of 1 mg intravenous (10 mL of 1:10 000 concentration solution).

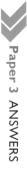

As an infusion at a rate of 0.04 to 0.4 micrograms·kg^{-1}·min^{-1}, it can be used in the treatment of critical illness with circulatory failure.

Adrenaline is also used in the treatment of open angle glaucoma as a 1% topical solution. In combination with local anaesthetic solutions, adrenaline is used at a concentration of either 1:80 000 or 1:200 000 solution as a local vasoconstrictor. Adrenaline is also used in nebulized or inhaled formulation.

Further reading

Resuscitation Council (UK). Emergency treatment of anaphylactic reactions. 2008. [Online] Available from: http://www.resus.org.uk/pages/reaction.pdf.

Sasada M, Smith S. *Drugs in Anaesthesia and Intensive Care*. 3rd ed. Oxford: Oxford University Press; 2003.

9A: True
9B: True
9C: True
9D: False
9E: True
A benzyl group is an unsaturated six-carbon ring. This means that the ring contains some C=C bonds. Suxamethonium is essentially two acetylcholine groups joined through their acetyl groups. It contains no carbon ring structure. The anticholinesterases, salicylic acids, opioids and local anaesthetic agents all contain a benzyl group.

Further reading

Peck TE, Hill SA, Williams M. *Pharmacology for Anaesthesia and Intensive Care*, 3rd ed. Cambridge: Cambridge University Press; 2009.

10A: True
10B: True
10C: False
10D: False
10E: True
Hepatotoxicity is caused by anti-metabolites (methotrexate, azathioprine), nitrosureas, cytotoxic antibiotics as well as the aforementioned drugs. Vinblastine, a plant alkaloid, tends to cause pulmonary and cardio toxicity. Bleomycin is well known to cause pulmonary toxicity and also causes nephrotoxicity and cardiotoxicity.

Further reading

Allan N, Siller C, Breen A. Anaesthetic implications of chemotherapy. *Contin Educ Anaesth Crit Care Pain*. 2012; 12(2): 52–56.

11A: True
11B: False
11C: True
11D: False
11E: False

Catecholamine is the term used to describe a chemical formulation consisting of a benzene ring with an –OH group at C3 and C4 ('catechol') and an amine side chain at C1 ('amine').

Adrenaline, noradrenaline and dopamine are the only naturally occurring catecholamines. The initial precursor is the amino acid phenylalanine. This is synthesized to tyrosine, DOPA, dopamine, noradrenaline and finally adrenaline by specific enzymes at each stage. Synthetic catecholamines include isoprenaline, dobutamine and dopexamine.

Further reading

Peck TE, Hill SA, Williams M. *Pharmacology for Anaesthesia and Intensive Care.* 3rd ed. Cambridge: Cambridge University Press; 2009.

12A: False
12B: True
12C: True
12D: True
12E: False

There are a number of models used for target-controlled infusions (TCI). Most are for use with propofol and include Marsh, Schüttler and White-Kenny, Schneider, Kataria and Paedfusor. The Minto model is designed for use with remifentanil. The Marsh model requires age to be entered but does not use it in its calculation. It merely prevents use of the algorithm in patients younger than 16 years of age. The Schneider model uses height, weight and sex to calculate lean body mass. Elderly patients have a lower central volume of distribution so require a relatively lower infusion rate for similar anaesthetic effect. In contrast children have a relatively higher central volume of distribution and require a higher infusion rate. There is a fourfold difference in the central compartment volume calculated by the Marsh and Schneider models; the Marsh model calculates the higher value. All the algorithms use three superimposed infusions: one at a constant rate to match drug elimination and two others as exponentially declining rates, which match drug removal from the central to peripheral compartments.

Further reading

Guarracino F, Lapolla F, Cariello C, Danella A, Doroni L, Baldassarri R, Boldrini A, Volpe ML. Target controlled infusion: TCI. *Minerva Anestesiol.* 2005; 71(6): 335–337.

13A: False
13B: True
13C: False
13D: True
13E: True

Vomiting is the forceful expulsion of gastric contents through the mouth. Nausea is the unpleasant sensation associated with the desire to vomit. The vomiting reflex consists of the following parts.

Afferents

- Visceral afferents: vagal afferents from the gastrointestinal tract mechano- and chemoreceptors (muscarinic acetylcholine receptors, visceral $5HT_3$ receptors)
- Vestibular afferents: stimulation of labyrinthine system is a potent stimulus for vomiting (muscarinic acetylcholine receptors)
- Chemoreceptor trigger zone (CTZ): lies in area postrema in floor of fourth ventricle; lies outside blood–brain barrier and cerebrospinal fluid so can detect blood-borne toxins (contains $5HT_3$ and D_2 dopaminergic receptors)
- Limbic system: emotional input to vomiting

The vomiting centre (VC) – Central coordination

The vomiting centre lies within the medulla of the brainstem. It is not really a discrete centre, it may include the:

- Dorsal and ventral respiratory groups
- Dorsal motor vagal nucleus
- Nucleus tractus solitaries
- Parvicellular reticular formation

It receives input from all afferents and sends efferent supply to the:

- Vagus nerves
- Phrenic nerves
- Spinal motor nerves supplying abdominal muscles

The vomiting reflex can be targeted pharmacologically at any point along this pathway.

Dopamine antagonists – Act at the VC, CTZ

- Phenothiazines are anti-psychotic drugs with a limited benefit in the treatment of nausea and vomiting due to their anti-D_2 actions. Drugs include chlorprpmazine and prochlorperazine.
- Domperidone is a D_2 receptor antagonist that does not cross the blood–brain barrier and therefore caused less extra-pyramidal side effects than phenothiazines but was withdrawn due to arrhythmias.
- Droperidol is a butyrophenone that antagonizes central D_2 receptors in the CTZ. However, it is not available in the United Kingdom.
- Metoclopramide is an antagonist at CTZ D_2 receptors but also has prokinetic effects on the stomach and has some anti-$5HT_3$ effects.

Anticholinergics – Act at the VC (input from vestibular system, visceral afferents)

- Hyoscine and atropine are tertiary amines and therefore able to cross the blood–brain barrier. Only hyoscine is useful as an antiemetic as it does not cause cardiovascular side effects.

Anti-serotonergics (anti-5HT$_3$) – Act at the CTZ and at peripheral visceral 5HT$_3$ receptors to the VC

- Ondansetron is a carbazole that acts as an antagonist at central and peripheral 5HT$_3$ receptors.

Antihistamines – Act at the VC

- Cyclizine is the most commonly used antihistamine antiemetic. It is an antagonist at H$_1$ receptors but also has anticholinergic effects.

Cannabinoids – Act at the VC

- Nabilone is a synthetic cannabinol that acts on cannabinoid receptors in the vomiting centre and is useful in chemotherapy-induced nausea and vomiting.

Neurokinin (NK$_1$) receptor antagonists – Act at the VC

- Selective neurokinin receptor antagonists such as aprepitant have been shown to have antiemetic activity by antagonizing neurokinin receptors in the nucleus tractus solitarius of the vomiting centre.

Further reading

Pierre S, Whelan R. Nausea and vomiting after surgery. *Contin Educ Anaesth Crit Care Pain*. 2013; 13(1): 23–27.

14A: False
14B: False
14C: True
14D: True
14E: False

Drugs are often metabolized within the body to form more water-soluble compounds that can be more easily excreted in the urine or bile. Occasionally this produces more active compounds as in the case of prodrugs such as enalapril.

There are two phases of metabolism. Phase 1 metabolism often occurs within the cytochrome P450 enzyme system of the liver. Phase 1 reactions include oxidation, reduction and hydrolysis.

However, members of the P450 family of enzymes are also present within the gut, lung, brain and kidney; phase 1 reactions can take place in these sites and also in other sites by other enzyme systems. Angiotensin converting enzyme (ACE) within the lung breaks down bradykinin and is responsible for metabolism of angiotensin-I to angiotensin-II. Monoamines such as adrenaline and noradrenaline are metabolized by mitochondrial monoamine oxidase and some drugs are metabolized within the cytoplasm.

Phase 2 metabolism: these reactions include conjugation reactions such as glucuronidation, sulphation and acetylation. They increase the water solubility of drugs, making them more readily excreted in bile or urine. Many drugs undergo phase 2 metabolism after phase 1 metabolism but some drugs only undergo phase 2 metabolism. This normally takes place in the endoplasmic reticulum of the liver, but also in other sites, such as the lung.

Some drugs enhance or inhibit the activity of the hepatic cytochrome P450 enzymes. This can alter plasma levels of other drugs also metabolized by the P450 system.

Hepatic Enzyme Inducers	Hepatic Enzyme Inhibitors
Glucocorticoids/Griseofulvin	Phenelzine
Phenobarbitone	Isoniazid
Phenytoin	Grapefruit juice
Rifampicin	Metronidazole
Inhalational anaesthetics	Erythromycin
Carbamazepine	Cimetidine
Ethanol (chronic)	Amiodarone
Smoking	Ketoconazole
	Ethanol (acute)
	Sulphonylureas

Further reading

Peck TE, Hill SA, Williams M. *Pharmacology for Anaesthesia and Intensive Care.* 3rd ed. Cambridge: Cambridge University Press; 2008. Chapter 2, p. 8–22.

15A: False
15B: True
15C: True
15D: False
15E: False

Phosphodiesterase (PDE) is an enzyme family of five isoenzymes that catalyze the hydrolysis of cyclic AMP (cAMP) and cyclic GMP (cGMP). This leads to a reduction of intracellular cAMP and cGMP levels.

Intracellular cAMP is a second messenger involved in many metabolic pathways. It is the final common pathway of a number of extracellular stimuli and causes protein kinase activation; in particular, protein kinase A activation. PDE III is found in cardiac muscle and vascular smooth muscle, and implicated in cardiovascular functioning.

Inhibition increases myocardial cAMP levels and therefore promotes intracellular calcium influx during the action potential, required for cardiac muscle contraction. This exerts a positive inotropic effect. In addition, it leads to vasodilatation.

Aminophylline is a non-selective PDE inhibitor that causes bronchodilation and improved diaphragm contractility and has mild positive inotropic and chronotropic effects.

Enoximone is a selective PDE III inhibitor, used in the treatment of acute-on-chronic heart failure, in low output states prior to cardiac transplant and during and after withdrawal of cardiopulmonary bypass. It increases cardiac output, left ventricular stroke volume and reduces systemic vascular resistance, pulmonary vascular resistance and right atrial pressure. It is metabolized in the liver to an active sulphoxide form and is excreted predominantly in this form in the urine.

Milrinone is also a selective PDE III inhibitor that works in a similar manner to enoximone but has been associated with increased mortality when used orally in severe heart failure.

Further reading

Feneck R. Phosphodiesterase inhibitors and the cardiovascular system. *Contin Educ Anaesth Crit Care Pain.* 2007; 7(6): 203–207.

Hasenfuss G, Teerlink JR. Cardiac inotropes: current agents and future directions. *Eur Heart J.* 2011; 32(15): 1838–1845.

16A: True
16B: True
16C: False
16D: True
16E: True

Suxamethonium is the only depolarizing neuromuscular blocking drug in clinical use. It has a chemical structure similar to acetylcholine (ACh); in fact it is a dicholine ester of succinic acid.

It binds to nicotinic ACh receptors at the neuromuscular junction in the same way as ACh but it is hydrolyzed at a slower rate and therefore prevents binding of ACh to the receptors. Suxamethonium is hydrolyzed by plasma cholinesterase (also known as pseudo-cholinesterase), present in the liver and plasma. Deficiency or polymorphisms in this enzyme can result in prolonged neuromuscular blockade.

On binding, suxamethonium induces an action potential in the motor neurone, resulting in muscle fasciculation initially, which commonly leads to postoperative myalgia, especially in young females.

Suxamethonium causes tachycardia following a single dose, but bradycardia may also occur, particularly with repeated doses and in the paediatric population, due to stimulation of muscarinic receptors at the sino-atrial node.

Suxamethonium is a potent trigger for malignant hyperpyrexia in susceptible individuals and may also cause severe anaphylactoid reactions. Suxamethonium causes a transient rise in serum potassium level (approximately 0.5 to 1.0 mmol·L^{-1}) and it should be used with caution in patients with renal impairment, or in patients with burns, paralysis or prolonged immobility, in whom it may precipitate dangerous hyperkalaemia and cardiac arrest due to the presence of extra-junctional acetylcholine receptors.

Further reading

Smith S, Scarth E, Sasada M. *Drugs in Anaesthesia and Intensive Care.* 4th ed. Oxford: Oxford University Press; 2011.

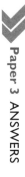

17A: False
17B: True
17C: False
17D: True
17E: True

The QT interval is a measure of the time taken for a cycle of ventricular depolarization and repolarization, and is measured as the time between the beginning of the electrocardiogram Q wave and the end of the T wave. It varies with heart rate and is therefore corrected to give the QTc. Prolongation of the QT interval can be due to genetic or acquired causes but is often due to a combination of a genetic predisposition and acquired factors. Prolongation of QT interval leads to impairment of ventricular repolarization, which can predispose to polymorphic ventricular tachycardia (torsade de pointes). Drugs that prolong QT interval include most volatile anaesthetic agents, amiodarone, flecainide, thiazides, phenothiazines, tricyclic antidepressants and suxamethonium. In addition, excessive stress can trigger torsades de pointes in patients with prolonged QT interval. Care must therefore be taken in administering general anaesthesia in such patients.

Further reading

Hunter JD, Sharma P, Rathi S. Long QT syndrome. *Contin Educ Anaesth Crit Care Pain.* 2008; 8(2): 67–70.

Peck TE, Hill SA, Williams M. *Pharmacology for Anaesthesia and Intensive Care.* 3rd ed. Cambridge: Cambridge University Press; 2008. Chapter 14, p. 228–245.

18A: True
18B: False
18C: False
18D: False
18E: True

Tachyarrhythmias may result from enhanced automaticity of cardiac myocytes outside the sino-atrial node, instability in membrane potential within ischaemic cells following myocardial infarction, or re-entry mechanisms. They are classified as supraventricular or ventricular tachyarrhythmias depending on their site of origin and are treated by differing methods.

The traditional Vaughan–Williams classification of anti-arrhythmic drugs classifies drugs by their mechanism of action into four classes. Class I includes drugs that delay conduction through fast sodium channels. They can be further classified according to their effect on the duration of the cardiac action potential refractory period (RP). Class II anti-arrhythmics act by inhibition of β-adrenoceptors, whereas class III anti-arrhythmics act by blocking conduction through potassium ion channels. Finally, class IV anti-arrhythmics are those that act on calcium channels, blocking their action.

Class I Anti-Arrhythmics	Class II Anti-Arrhythmics	Class III Anti-Arrhythmics	Class IV Anti-Arrhythmics
Block Na⁺ Channels	Beta-Blockers	Block K⁺ Channels	Ca²⁺ Channel Blockers
Prolong RP (Ia)	Acebutolol	Amiodarone	Diltiazem
Disopyramide	Atenolol	Sotalol	Verapamil
Procainamide	Bisoprolol	Bretylium	
Quinidine	Carvedilol	Azimilide	
	Esmolol		
Shortens RP (Ib)	Metoprolol		
Lidocaine	Propranolol		
Mexilitine	Timolol		
Phenytoin	Sotalol		
No effect on RP (Ic)			
Flecainide			
Propafenone			

Note: RP = refractory period.

The Vaughan–Williams classification has limitations including the lack of classification of a number of commonly used drugs such as digoxin. It may therefore be more helpful to consider anti-arrhythmic drugs by the type of tachyarrhythmia they are used to treat: supraventricular, ventricular or both.

Supraventricular Arrhythmias	Ventricular Arrhythmias	Both
Digoxin	Lidocaine	Amiodarone
Adenosine	Mexilitine	Flecainide
Verapamil		Disopyramide
Quinidine		Propafenone
β-blockers (except sotalol)		Procainamide
		Sotalol

Further reading

Singh BN. Current antiarrhythmic drugs: an overview of mechanisms of action and potential clinical utility. *J Cardiovasc Electrophysiol*. 1999 Feb; 10(2): 283–301.

19A: True
19B: True
19C: True
19D: False
19E: True
Drug metabolism occurs within the body to form more water-soluble compounds that can be more easily excreted in the urine or bile. Occasionally this produces more active compounds as in the case of prodrugs such as enalapril.

There are two phases of metabolism: Phase 1 and phase 2 reactions.

Phase 1 reactions include oxidation, reduction and hydrolysis. These can occur within the lung, mitochondrial monoamine oxidase, and within the cytoplasm but most often occur within the cytochrome P450 enzyme system of the liver. Members of the P450 enzyme family are also present in the gut, lung, brain and kidney. There are many different isoforms within this family, each of which is responsible for the metabolism of different compounds. Genetic polymorphisms within these isoenzymes can affect the metabolism of drugs such as codeine, metabolized by the CYP2D6 isoform, or sevoflurane, metabolized by the 2E1 isoform.

Other phase 1 metabolism affected by genetic polymorphisms includes drugs hydrolyzed by the enzyme plasma cholinesterase. Single amino acid substitutions are responsible for four alleles conferring altered enzyme activity and reduced metabolism of drugs such as suxamethonium.

Phase 2 reactions are synthetic reactions increasing the water solubility of compounds. They include conjugation reactions, such as glucuronidation and acetylation, and occur mainly within the liver. Acetylation is a hepatic phase 2 pathway that can be affected by genetic polymorphisms, resulting in fast or slow acetylation. This can affect the metabolism of drugs such as isoniazid and hydralazine.

Further reading

Iohom G, Fitzgerald D, Cunningham AJ. Principles of pharmacogenetics: implications for the anaesthetist. *Br J Anaesth.* 2004; 93(3): 440–450.

20A: False
20B: False
20C: True
20D: False
20E: False
Antimicrobial agents act to either kill microorganisms (bactericidal) or suppress their activity and growth (bacteriostatic). They can have their action in three main areas: interfering with bacterial cell wall synthesis or integrity, inhibition of bacterial protein synthesis or interruption of DNA synthesis.

Penicillins (amoxicillin, benzylpenicillin) act by inhibiting synthesis of the bacterial cell wall. They are bactericidal but rarely destroy bacteria to the point of eradication. This can be achieved by combining them with another bactericidal drug such as gentamicin. Glycopeptide antimicrobials, such as teicoplanin and vancomycin, also act on the cell wall of bacteria preventing peptidoglycan formation and are bactericidal.

Gentamicin is an aminoglycoside antibiotic, a class of drugs that act by irreversibly binding to the 30S subunit of the bacterial ribosome, preventing initiation of ribosomal protein synthesis and causing mRNA misreading. This results in cell death. Macrolide antimicrobials act in a similar fashion by binding to, and inhibiting the action of, the other 50S ribosomal subunit. Macrolides include erythromycin, clarithromycin and azithromycin. They can have bacteriostatic or bactericidal action depending on their plasma concentration.

Lincosamides, such as clindamycin, also act to interfere with the 50S subunit but are bacteriostatic in their action. Quinolones, such as ciprofloxacin and nalidixic acid, lead to cell death by inhibition of DNA gyrase, preventing DNA supercoiling. Metronidazole acts by breaking bacterial DNA strands and inhibiting nucleic acid synthesis.

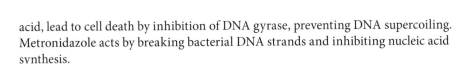

Further reading

Varley AJ, Sule J, Absalom AR. Principles of antibiotic therapy. *Contin Educ Anaesth Crit Care Pain.* 2009; 9(6): 184–188.

21A: False
21B: True
21C: False
21D: False
21E: False
Electrical thermometers include the resistance thermometer, thermistor, thermocouple and infrared thermometer.

Resistance thermometer

- Components: platinum wire, battery, ammeter (which measures electrical current).
- Mechanism: a current is conducted from the battery along the platinum wire. Platinum will have varying resistance to current flow depending on the temperature. The magnitude of current conducted is measured and displayed by the ammeter. The relationship between change in resistance of a conductor and temperature is linear.
- The resistance thermometer is a rapidly responsive device but is relatively insensitive. The addition of a Wheatstone bridge increases sensitivity.

Thermistor

- Components: small bead of a semi-conductor metal oxide.
- Mechanism: the semi-conductor metal oxide exhibits an exponential decline in resistance with increasing temperature.
- The thermistor is used with a Wheatstone bridge, so is highly sensitive as well as cheap and robust.
- Calibration is required as the system is prone to drift with time.
- The system is sensitive to severe changes in temperature, for example, heat sterilization.

Thermocouple

- Components: two dissimilar metals (commonly copper and constantin) in a circuit.
- Mechanism: the Seebeck effect, where at a junction between two dissimilar metals, the voltage present will be proportional to the temperature. A second junction completes the circuit and is kept at a constant temperature to act as a reference junction.
- The device is simple, cheap, small and responds to a wide temperature range.

Infrared

- Principle: the Stefan–Boltzmann law describes the behaviour of a perfect black body, which will absorb energies at all wavelengths then emit energy at a wavelength depending on the body's temperature. A cold body will emit no light (and hence will appear black). The total emissive power (E) of the body is proportional to the fourth power of the body's absolute temperature (T).

$$\text{Stefan–Boltzmann principle: } E = \varepsilon \, \sigma \, A \, T^4$$

where

E = emissive power of the body

ε = emissive efficiency (1 for a black body, near 0 for a silvered body)

σ = Stefan's constant

A = area

T = absolute temperature

- Mechanism: the infrared ear probe is inserted into the ear canal. A beam of infrared radiation is directed onto the tympanic membrane and the amount of infrared emitted is detected by a sensor.
- This system is non-invasive, rapid and gives a core temperature reading.
- It is worth noting that a 'black body' is a hypothetical model.

Further reading

Sullivan G, Edmondson C. Heat and temperature. *Contin Educ Anaesth Crit Care Pain*. 2008; 8(3): 104–107.

22A: True
22B: True
22C: False
22D: True
22E: False

The heat and moisture exchange device (HME) is a passive humidification device commonly used in anaesthesia and intensive care.

- Components: plastic housing, two ports (15 and 22 mm outer diameters), a port for oxygen tubing/gas sampling, a highly folded hygrophobic medium (composed of ceramic fibre, paper, cellulose, corrugated aluminium, foam or stainless steel fibre).
- Mechanism of action: on expiration, exhaled gas passes through the humidifier, where exhaled water vapour condenses on the cool medium. On inspiration, the condensed water evaporates, warming and humidifying inspired gas.
- Factors affecting performance: time (the device takes up to 20 minutes to start working efficiently), the water vapour content of patients' respiratory gas, the fresh gas flow rates (the device is less efficient at higher flow rates) and the temperature of the respiratory gas.
- Advantages: the HME device is compact, inexpensive and reasonably efficient (achieving a relative humidity of 60–70%, gas temperature of 29–34°C and an

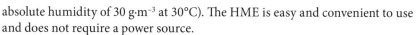

absolute humidity of 30 g·m⁻³ at 30°C). The HME is easy and convenient to use and does not require a power source.

- Disadvantages: the HME produces resistance to gas flow (0.1–2 cmH$_2$O) and may obstruct with mucous, foreign bodies, water accumulation and by expansion of the hygrophobic medium when saturated. The HME is designed for single patient use, for a maximum duration of 24 hours; two-way gas flow is necessary and it is less efficient with larger tidal volumes.

Further reading

Al Shaikh B, Stacey S. *Essentials of Anaesthetic Equipment.* 3rd ed. Philadelphia: Elsevier Health Sciences; 2007.

Wilkes AR. Humidification: its importance and delivery. *Contin Educ Anaesth Crit Care Pain.* 2001; 1(2): 40–43.

23A: True
23B: False
23C: True
23D: False
23E: False

The Severinghaus CO$_2$ electrode is used to measure the partial pressure of carbon dioxide in a sample of blood. The system is based on the pH electrode, where hydrogen ions are produced in proportion to the partial pressure of CO$_2$.

$$CO_2 + H_2O \rightleftharpoons H_2CO_3 \rightleftharpoons H^+ + HCO_3^-$$

Components

Two electrodes:

- Glass electrode: consists of a hydrogen sensitive glass, covered in a nylon mesh and coated with a thin film of sodium bicarbonate solution (which acts as a buffer).
- Reference electrode: consists of silver/silver chloride in a potassium chloride electrolyte solution with water.

Mechanism of action

Both the electrodes are contained within a membrane that is in contact with the blood sample. The membrane is permeable to CO$_2$ but impermeable to red blood cells, hydrogen ions (H$^+$), plasma and bicarbonate (HCO$_3^-$).

CO$_2$ diffuses through the membrane into the nylon mesh, where it combines with water to make H$^+$ and HCO$_3^-$ ions via carbonic acid (see earlier). The glass electrode measures the change in H$^+$ tension and therefore partial pressure of CO$_2$ (pCO$_2$) is measured.

Advantages

Accurate, stable.

Disadvantages

The device requires regular calibration to ensure accuracy. The measurement is slow, as the CO_2 must diffuse through the membrane and dissociate before a measurement can be made. The process usually takes 2 to 3 minutes; however, it can be sped up by the addition of carbonic anhydrase. Accuracy of the electrode also requires the maintenance of a constant temperature, and disintegration of the membrane will lead to inaccurate readings.

Further reading

Al Shaikh B, Stacey S. *Essentials of Anaesthetic Equipment.* 3rd ed. Philadelphia: Elsevier Health Sciences; 2007.

Davis PD, Kenny GNC. *Basic Physics and Measurement in Anaesthesia.* 5th ed. Oxford: Butterworth-Heinemann; 2003.

Langton JA, Hutton A. Respiratory gas analysis. *Contin Educ Anaesth Crit Care Pain.* 2009; (9)1: 19–23.

24A: False
24B: True
24C: False
24D: False
24E: False

Electric shock occurs when an individual becomes part of a circuit. The degree of damage due to electrocution depends on the current size, the path through the individual, the type of current (AC or DC), the duration of contact, the current density and the frequency of current. The most lethal frequency is mains frequency (50 Hz), which is used for mains supply in the United Kingdom, as it is easily generated at high voltages and transmitted easily along power cables.

At 50 Hz alternating current:

- 1 mA will cause tingling
- 5 mA will cause pain
- 8 mA will cause burns
- 15 mA will cause tonic muscle contraction of flexor muscles
- 50 mA will cause respiratory arrest and severe pain
- 75–100 mA will cause ventricular fibrillation

Further reading

Al Shaikh B, Stacey S. *Essentials of Anaesthetic Equipment.* 3rd ed. Edinburgh: Churchill Livingstone; 2006.

Boumphrey S, Langton JA. Electrical safety in the operating theatre. *Contin Educ Anaesth Crit Care Pain.* 2003; (3)1: 10–14.

25A: True
25B: False
25C: True
25D: False
25E: False

Reusable anaesthetic equipment requires decontamination between patients to prevent transmission of disease. Decontamination is a process that removes or destroys contaminants. It is usually cleaning followed by disinfection and/or sterilization. The method and level of decontamination required depends on the nature of the equipment and patient exposure. Equipment can be classified according to risk of transmission of infection:

- Critical items: those that breach sterile tissue or blood vessels (e.g. surgical instruments, catheters). They must be sterilized.
- Semi-critical: those in contact with mucous membranes or intact skin (e.g. laryngoscopes, breathing circuits). They require at least high-level disinfection.
- Non-critical: those that come into contact with healthy skin but not mucous membranes (e.g. blood pressure cuffs). They require cleaning.

Different levels of decontamination are described next.

Cleaning is the physical removal of foreign material; it reduces bio-burden but does not necessarily destroy infectious agents:

- Point of care decontamination of non-critical items: usually washing with cool water and detergent (<45°C).

Disinfection is the elimination of most pathogenic agents but excluding bacterial spores:

- Chemical disinfectants
  - Low level: kill most vegetative bacteria and viruses (e.g. alcohols and sodium hypochlorite (bleach)
  - High level: those that kill spores (e.g. glutaraldehyde, sodium peroxide, chlorine)
- Pasteurization: hot water >77°C for at least 30 minutes.

Sterilization is the complete destruction of all forms of microbial life.

- Steam
- Glutaraldehyde
- Ethylene oxide
- Gas plasma
- Prion protein transmission is still not well understood, therefore single-use instruments are recommended for those suspected of carrying variant CJD

Further reading

Sabir N, Ramachandran V. Decontamination of anaesthetic equipment. *Contin Educ Anaesth Crit Care Pain.* 2004; 4(4): 103–106.

26A: False
26B: True
26C: False
26D: False
26E: False

Mechanically ventilating a patient's lungs can be achieved using either negative or positive pressure, although positive pressure ventilation is the most commonly used in current medical practice. During positive pressure ventilation, sufficient pressure must be generated by the ventilator to overcome the elastic recoil of the lungs and the chest wall, as well as the resistance created by the airways.

There are a number of ways to classify ventilators:

- Methods of pressure generation: pressure generators, flow generators
- According to cycling: intermittent ventilation is said to 'cycle' between both inspiratory and expiratory phases. Each of these phases can be controlled according to volume, time, pressure and flow.
- According to application in clinical practice:
  - Mechanical thumbs
  - Intermittent blowers
  - Minute volume dividers
  - Bag squeezers

Mechanical thumb type ventilators utilize a pressurized gas source to provide a continuous flow. By occluding the open end of a T-piece breathing system, the flow is diverted to the patient's lungs until the end is opened again. This system is wasteful of gas and is therefore only suitable for paediatric and neonatal anaesthesia.

Minute volume dividers use pressurized gas fed into a continually pressurized reservoir, which alternately has gas either diverted to or away from it, and fills (during expiration) or discharges the reservoir volume to the patient (inspiration).

Bag squeezers are the most commonly used form of ventilator during anaesthesia. The bag or bellows is squeezed pneumatically by pressure of driving gas fed into a space between the bellows and its casing.

Intermittent blowers are driven by a pressurized source of gas that feeds into a low compliance internal pathway, using either pneumatic oscillation or proportional flow valves to control the size and rate of tidal volumes. These are the most common type of ventilators used in intensive care settings.

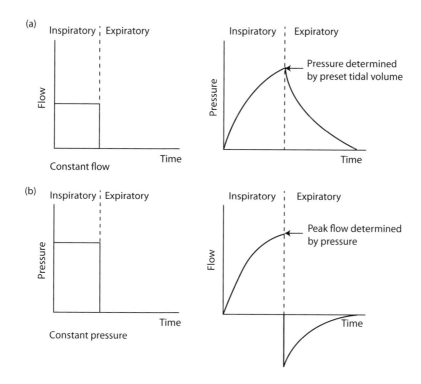

Further reading

Davey AJ, Diba A. *Ward's Anaesthetic Equipment*. 5th ed. Philadelphia: Elsevier Saunders; 2005. Chapter 11, p. 241–265.

27A: False
27B: True
27C: False
27D: True
27E: True

Sidestream capnography draws a gas sample from the expiratory limb of the breathing circuit, from as close to the patient and possible. Gas is drawn at a flow rate of 150–200 ml·min^{-1}. This is carried by a Teflon-coated tube of internal diameter 1–2 mm. Teflon is used as it is impermeable to CO_2 and does not react with volatile anaesthetic agents. The system incorporates a moisture trap to prevent water from blocking the tube. The gas sample is carried to an infrared photospectrometer, where it is analyzed. The exhaust post then returns the gas either back to the circuit or to be scavenged. Advantages of sidestream capnography are easy connection, measurement of multiple gases, minimal dead space, it can be used in non-intubated patients and it is a robust and lightweight device. A portable system is also available.

Mainstream capnography incorporates a sampling chamber within the breathing system. This contains a sapphire windowed chamber through which gas flows in order to avoid water condensation on the window. It is heated to 41°C and the analyzer sits over the chamber (you are aware of this as it takes time to warm up before giving a reading). Advantages of this device are the avoidance of a transit time, lack of a sampling line, which avoids loss of gas, and it is a simpler device, which does not require regular calibration. Disadvantages are that it is currently only used for CO_2 analysis, it is bulky and fragile, and damage to the window is common. There are additional risks associated with the heating device and burns are possible. Mainstream analyzers are more commonly used in paediatric anaesthesia.

Further reading

Langton JA, Hutton A. Respiratory gas analysis. *Contin Educ Anaesth Crit Care Pain*. 2009; 9(1): 19–23.

28A: True
28B: True
28C: False
28D: False
28E: True

Intravenous giving sets are designed to administer fluid and blood products. The adult giving set is composed of a clear plastic tube with a spike at one end for insertion into the bag of fluid and a Luer lock adapter for attachment to a cannula at the other end. The controller chamber permits a drop size of 20 drops of clear fluid per millilitre and 15 drops of blood per millilitre.

Blood giving sets are of larger diameter and incorporate a filter of 150 micrometre mesh, which sits in a chamber with a plastic ball float. Platelets can be administered through a blood giving set, provided this has not already been used for other blood products.

The paediatric giving set has a burette, with 1 mL gradations to allow accurate measurement of fluid volumes. The drop size is 60 drops of clear fluid per millilitre. The addition of 0.2 micrometre filters to paediatric giving sets reduces the incidence of thrombophlebitis related to infusions.

Further reading

Al-Shaikh B, Stacey S. *Essentials of Anaesthetic Equipment*. 2nd ed. Edinburgh: Harcourt Publishers Limited; 2002.

Smith T, Pinnock C, Lin T. *Fundamentals of Anaesthesia*. 3rd ed. Cambridge: Cambridge University Press; 2009.

29A: False
29B: False
29C: True
29D: False
29E: True

Volumetric pumps, such as those used for epidural infusions, are best used for infusions requiring medium to high flow rates greater than 5 ml·hr⁻¹. They have variable short-term accuracy and are better for delivering a set volume rather than flow. Volumetric pumps have an alarm system that detects occlusion or air in the infusion line when the pump door is open and the battery is low. These pumps are accurate to within 5 to 10%. There are four types of volumetric pumps: drip counters (which work with gravity and a photoelectric drip rate counter), peristaltic, rotary and piston pump mechanisms.

Further reading

Al-Shaikh B, Stacey S. *Essentials of Anaesthetic Equipment*. 2nd ed. Edinburgh: Churchill Livingstone; 2002.

30A: True
30B: False
30C: True
30D: True
30E: True

Capacitance is the property of a device that enables it to store electrical charge. A capacitor consists of two conducting plates, which are separated by thin layers of insulating material (the dielectric). When a voltage is applied across the plates, an initial surge of current moves the charge onto the plates. When the plates are fully charged, no further current flows. The amount of charge stored depends on the size of the capacitance, which is measured in farads (F). The capacitance is influenced by the size of the capacitor plates (the greater the plate area, the greater the capacitance), the separation of the plates (the greater the distance, the lower the capacitance) and the dielectric material used. The charge stored in a capacitor is calculated by:

$$\text{Charge (Q)} = \text{Capacitance (C)} \times \text{Voltage (V)}$$

In a circuit, AC signals are able to pass as electrostatic forces between the capacitor plates transmit the constantly changing AC current. DC signals are blocked as there is no direct contact between the plates. The impedance of a capacitor is inversely related to the frequency of the current; hence capacitors have higher impedance to low frequency current. Capacitors are used in electrosurgical equipment as isolating devices, as they have high impedance to mains frequency.

Inductors have low resistance to DC signals and high reactance to AC signals.

Further reading

Boumphrey S, Langton JA. Electrical safety in the operating theatre. *Contin Educ Anaesth Crit Care Pain*. 2003; 3(1): 10–14.

Davis PD. *Basic Physics and Measurement in Anaesthesia*. 5th ed. Oxford: Butterworth-Heinemann; 2003.

Smith T, Pinnock C, Lin T. *Fundamentals of Anaesthesia*. 3rd ed. Cambridge: Cambridge University Press; 2009.

31A: False
31B: True
31C: False
31D: False
31E: True
The basic quantities of electricity are current, voltage and resistance.

The ampere (A) is the unit of electrical current, not the coulomb (unit of charge). Current is the flow of electrical charge and is a measure of the amount of electrons flowing past a point in a circuit per unit time. The SI unit of electrical current is the ampere, named after André-Marie Ampère, a French mathematician and physicist. One ampere is the flow of 1 coulomb of charge past a point in a circuit each second. The coulomb is a unit of electrical charge and is equivalent to the charge carried in 6.24×10^{18} electrons.

Voltage, or potential difference, is the electrical force that drives the current. One volt (V) is the potential difference between two points on a conducting wire carrying 1 ampere of current, between which 1 watt of power is dissipated. It is also equal to 1 joule of energy per coulomb of charge.

The resistance determines the amount of current when a given voltage is applied across a conductor. If the resistance is low, then for a given voltage the current will be higher and vice versa. The resistance of a conductor depends upon the material and its shape. A long wire has a higher resistance than a short wire, and a thick wire has a lower resistance than a thin wire. The unit for resistance is the volt·amp^{-1}, called an ohm (Ω).

Further reading

Singh S, Ingham R, Golding J. Basics of electricity for anaesthetists. *Contin Educ Anaesth Crit Care Pain*. 2011; 11(6): 224–228.

32A: True
32B: False
32C: True
32D: True
32E: False
The monitoring of respiratory gases is now standard practice in theatre, ICU and during patient transfer. In the AAGBI guidelines of 2007 the following are regarded as essential components during anaesthesia: oxygen analyzer with an audible alarm; a carbon dioxide analyzer; and a vapour analyzer for use with volatile anaesthetics. The measuring of ambient anaesthetic agent concentrations falls under the remit of COSHH standards.

Further reading

Association of Anaesthetists of Great Britain and Ireland (AAGBI). *Recommendations for Standards of Monitoring during Anaesthesia and Recovery*. 4th ed. 2007. [Online] Available from: http://www.aagbi.org/publications/guidelines/docs/standardsofmonitoring07.pdf.

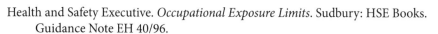

Health and Safety Executive. *Occupational Exposure Limits*. Sudbury: HSE Books. Guidance Note EH 40/96.

Langton JA, Hutton A. Respiratory gas analysis. *Contin Educ Anaesth Crit Care Pain*. 2009; 9: 19–23.

33A: False
33B: False
33C: True
33D: True
33E: False

There are fewer complications with non-invasive blood pressure measurement than with invasive. However, there have been reports of nerve damage occurring with repeated inflation of the cuff, particularly with the ulnar nerve at the elbow. The first time the cuff inflates the pressure is very high and is often painful for the patient, particularly if the cuff is on the calf. For the cuff to read accurately, it should have no external pressure applied to it. Therefore, when the patient is in the lateral position the cuff should be on the uppermost arm. Measurement can be difficult in the presence of arrhythmias, particularly atrial fibrillation. Measurement also tends to be more inaccurate than invasive techniques when the blood pressure is low.

Further reading

Ward M, Langton J. Blood pressure measurement. *Contin Educ Anaesth Crit Care Pain*. 2007; 7: 122–126.

34A: True
34B: False
34C: True
34D: False
34E: True

True positive (TP): the patient has the disease and the test is positive
False positive (FP): the patient does not have the disease but the test is positive
True negative (TN): the patient does not have the disease and the test is negative
False negative (FN): the patient has the disease but the test is negative
Sensitivity (SE) refers to the ability of a clinical test to correctly identify those with the disease.
Specificity (SP) refers to the ability of a clinical test to correctly identify those without the disease.
Positive predictive value (PPV) answers the question: how likely is it that this patient has the disease given the test is positive?
Negative predictive value (NPV) answers the question: how likely is it that this patient does not have the disease given the test is negative?

	As Determined by Gold Standard	
	Disease	Disease
Disease Test ⊕	TP	FP
Disease Test ⊖	FN	TN

$$SE = TP/(TP + FN) \times 100$$
$$SP = TN/(TN + FP) \times 100$$
$$PPV = TP/(TP + FP) \times 100$$
$$NPV = TN/(TN + FN) \times 100$$

Further reading

Lalkhen A, McCluskey A. Clinical tests: sensitivity and specificity. *Contin Educ Anaesth Crit Care Pain*. 2008; 8: 221–223.

35A: True
35B: False
35C: True
35D: True
35E: True
Ether or diethyl ether is a flammable hydrocarbon. In air it does not ignite easily and burns slowly. Ether exhibits the phenomena of a cool flame. When present in concentrations of 20–35% in air it can be ignited by an ignition temperature as little as 200°C. This flame can be difficult to see and detect, especially since ether is heavier than air and sinks to the floor. It can serve as an ignition source for a potentially explosive mixture of ether and oxygen.

The normal ignition temperature for other inflammable anaesthetic agents is 400–500°C. The volatile anaesthetic agents such as isoflurane, sevoflurane and desflurane are not inflammable; neither is halothane.

Ethyl chloride is very flammable and explosive in oxygen or nitrous oxide. Vaseline® is a trade name for a form of petroleum jelly. When gases are pressurized quickly there can be heat generated. This can cause ignition of a lubricant if it consists of a flammable material.

Further reading

Busato GA. Fires and explosions in the operating room. *Update in Anaesthesia*, [Online] 2008: 190–193. Available from: www.worldanaesthesia.org.

36A: False
36B: False
36C: False
36D: True
36E: True
There are a number of lung volumes that represent how much air is present in the lungs at different points in the breathing cycle. Lung capacities are the sum of a number of different lung volumes. All lung volumes can be measured by a simple spirometer except the residual volume (RV) and hence the functional residual capacity (FRC), the sum of the RV and the expiratory reserve volume. To measure the RV and hence the FRC we can use either the helium dilution technique or a body plethysmograph. The dilution technique works when using helium because it is almost insoluble in blood. A drawback of this technique is that the helium can

only be diluted in the air in the lungs that can be ventilated. If there is significant air trapping then the helium will not be diluted in these portions. Hence this technique is not very accurate in those patients with obstructive airway diseases. A more accurate technique in these cases is to use the body plethysmograph, which utilizes Boyle's law to calculate the lung volume by detecting a pressure change in an airtight box. When using the helium technique the patient is connected to the spirometer at the end of a normal breath to ensure the FRC is being measured and not other lung volumes.

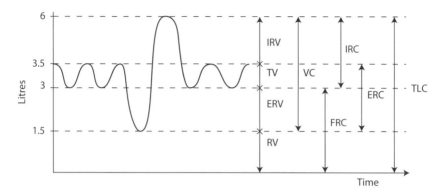

Abbreviations: IRV = Inspiratory Reserve Volume, TV = Tidal Volume, ERV = Expiratory Reserve Volume, RV = Residual Volume, VC = Vital Capacity, IRC = Inspiratory Reserve Capacity, ERC = Expiratory Reserve Capacity, FRC = Functional Residual Capacity, TLC = Total Lung Capacity

Further reading

West JB. *Respiratory Physiology: The Essentials*. 9th ed. Philadelphia: Lippincott Williams & Wilkins; 2011.

37A: False
37B: True
37C: False
37D: True
37E: False

The statistical test used to analyze data needs to be matched to the data type. Data may be qualitative or quantitative. After this split the distribution of the data needs to be assessed.

Normally distributed data from two groups is analyzed using the Student's *t*-test ('Student' was the pen name of WS Gosset who developed the test to compare the quality of stout while working at the Guinness brewery in Dublin). Non-normally distributed data from two groups is compared using the Mann–Whitney U-test.

If there are multiple groups then normally distributed data uses the analysis of variance or ANOVA, and non-normally distributed data the Kruskal–Wallis test. The chi-squared test is used to compare the observed frequency against the expected frequency in qualitative data.

Further reading

McCluskey A, Lalkhen AG. Statistics III: probability and statistical tests. *Contin Educ Anaesth Crit Care Pain.* 2007; 7(5): 167–170.

38A: False
38B: False
38C: True
38D: False
38E: False

In a measuring system, when the frequency of the waveform being measured coincides with the inherent frequency of the system then resonance will occur. This may distort the signal. The natural frequency of an arterial pressure monitoring system should be above 40 Hz to minimize resonance. Damping refers to the phenomenon where the rate of change between the patient and the pressure transducer is slowed down. Causes of damping include soft tubing, occlusion of the artery, a bubble or a soft cannula. Damping can be optimal where there is rapid change in signal with a small overshoot. Critical damping exists where there is no overshoot but the system is slow to respond. Overdamping exists where there is no overshoot but the response is so slow that it is inaccurate. Underdamping leads to resonance and overshoot.

The following are the respective values for damping factor: optimal, 0.7; critical, 1.0; underdamped, <0.7; and overdamped >1.0.

Further reading

Ward M, Langton J. Blood pressure measurement. *Contin Educ Anaesth Crit Care Pain.* 2007; 7: 122–126.

39A: True
39B: False
39C: True
39D: False
39E: True

A Bain circuit is a coaxial Mapleson D circuit that consists of an inner tube, which carries the fresh gas flow (FGF) to the patient end of the system, and an outer tube, which carries waste gases away from the patient.

During spontaneous ventilation:

- Inspiration: initially just FGF at first breath.
- Expiration: exhaled gas mixes with FGF and passes into reservoir bag, until full. The excess leaves via the adjustable pressure limiting (APL) valve.
- Expiratory pause: FGF displaces some of FGF/alveolar gas mixture out through the APL valve.
- Subsequent inspiration: initially stored fresh gas followed by mixture of FGF and exhaled gas in outer tube.

During controlled ventilation:

- Inspiration: at first bag squeeze, FGF entering system delivered to patient as well as fresh gas stored in outer tube. Some gas from reservoir lost through APL valve.
- Expiration: exhaled gas mixes with FGF and refills empty reservoir bag until full. The rest leaves via the APL valve.
- Expiratory pause: FGF replaces some of FGF/alveolar gas mixture out through APL.
- Subsequent inspiration: gas delivered to patient is continued FGF, plus fresh gas from outer tube, plus some exhaled gas left in outer tube. Some waste gas from reservoir bag is lost through the APL valve.

To prevent rebreathing:

- During controlled ventilation
  - FGF of at least alveolar ventilation
- During spontaneous ventilation
  - FGF of at least two to three times patient's minute ventilation

Mapleson A

Mapleson D

Mapleson B

Mapleson E

Mapleson C

Mapleson F

Further reading

Davey AJ, Diba A. *Ward's Anaesthetic Equipment*. 5th ed. Philadelphia: Elsevier Saunders; 2005. Chapter 2, p. 12–13.

40A: False
40B: True
40C: True
40D: False
40E: False
Mathematical functions allow relationships between different factors to be expressed in a logical and precise way and can allow us to simplify biological processes and design models to predict behaviour and activity.

A mathematical function describes the way in which one variable is affected by another. For example the way in which variable y is dependent on the variable x, can be expressed as $y = f(x)$.

The simplest form of relationship is known as a *linear relationship*:

- Can be plotted as a straight line on a graph of x vs. y
- Can be expressed as $y = mx + c$, where m is the gradient of the line, and c is the point at which it crosses the y axis

Inverse relationships exist when the increase in one variable results in a decrease in the corresponding variable, for example in the hyperbolic function, where $y = 1/x$.

Exponential functions involve one variable related to a number raised to a power. For example $y = b^x$. In this case, b is known as the base number. In an exponential relationship, the rate of change of a variable depends on the value of the variable at that time.

Logarithmic functions essentially result in the reflection of the function in the line $y = x$. They are useful in rearranging functions as they follow a number of rules:

- $\text{Log}(AB) = \text{Log } A + \text{Log } B$
- $\text{Log}(A/B) = \text{Log } A - \text{Log } B$
- $\text{Log}(b^x) = x \log b$

Taking logarithms of both sides of the exponential equation can allow it to be converted to a straight line, with the benefits that data can be much more easily extrapolated.

Further reading

Ercole A, Roe P. Mathematical relationships in anaesthesia and intensive care medicine. *Contin Educ Anaesth Crit Care Pain.* 2011; 11(2): 50–55.

41A: False
41B: True
41C: True
41D: True
41E: True
Chloride is the most abundant extracellular anion, with a normal plasma concentration of 95 to 105 mmol·L^{-1}. It has important roles in maintaining acid–base balance, as well as in renal tubular function and production of gastric

acid. Chloride buffers in a number of ways. It is transported into the cells of the proximal convoluted tubule in exchange for organic ions such as formate, facilitating transport of hydrogen ions into the tubular lumen where they can be excreted. Chloride moves into erythrocytes in exchange for bicarbonate ions as the 'chloride shift' (or Hamburger effect), which maintains electrical neutrality following HCO_3^- formation in carbon dioxide transportation. Chloride ions also contribute to the 'strong ion difference', determined by subtracting the concentrations of the major plasma anions (chloride and lactate) from the sum of the major plasma cations (sodium, potassium, calcium and magnesium). This strong ion difference contributes to body hydrogen ion concentration.

Further reading

Lote CJ. *Principles of Renal Physiology*. 5th ed. New York: Springer; 2012.

Rassam SS, Counsel DJ. Perioperative electrolyte and fluid balance. *Contin Educ Anaesth Crit Care Pain*. 2005; 5(5): 157–160.

42A: False
42B: True
42C: False
42D: False
42E: True

The human kidneys are paired organs, situated in the retroperitoneum, that are responsible for urine formation, regulation of body water, sodium and other electrolyte balance as well as having an endocrine function. The kidneys receive 20–25% of cardiac output at rest, providing 500 ml per 100 g renal tissue per minute. The blood supply is not distributed evenly between the renal medulla and the cortex. Ninety-nine percent of blood flow is to the cortex, where the majority of nephrons are located; the remaining 1% flows to the medulla. Even within the medulla, the blood flow to the outer medulla is greater (50 ml·100 g^{-1}·min^{-1}) than that to the inner medulla (20 ml·100 g^{-1}·min^{-1}). Renal blood flow can be calculated after determining renal plasma flow, which equates to clearance of para-aminohippuric acid (PAH). Plasma describes the proportion of blood not containing red blood cells (i.e. [1 – haematocrit] × 100); therefore, renal blood flow can be determined using renal plasma flow and the haematocrit.

Further reading

Lote CJ. *Principles of Renal Physiology*. 5th ed. New York: Springer; 2012.

Stewart P. Physiology of the kidney. *Update in Anaesthesia*. 1998; 9(6): 1–3.

43A: True
43B: False
43C: False
43D: True
43E: False

Functional residual capacity (FRC) is the sum of the residual volume (RV) and the expiratory reserve volume (ERV). It is the volume remaining in the lungs at the end of expiration during normal tidal breathing. Normal FRC lies on the steepest part of the lung compliance curve, and is also associated with minimal pulmonary vascular resistance. The volume of FRC is normally approximately 2500 ml in an adult male (1800 ml in an adult female) but is reduced in conditions that displace the diaphragm cephalad, such as pregnancy or abdominal distension, as well as those that reduce RV, such as fibrotic lung disease or restrictive chest wall defects. In addition, lying supine will reduce the FRC as does general anaesthesia. Obstructive lung diseases in contrast, such as asthma and emphysema, will increase FRC. FRC is not affected by age, although closing capacity (CC) increases with age.

Further reading

West JB. *Respiratory Physiology: The Essentials.* 8th ed. Philadelphia: Lippincott Williams & Wilkins; 2008.

Wild M, Alagesan K. PEEP and CPAP. *Contin Educ Anaesth Crit Care Pain.* 2001; 1(3): 89–92.

44A: False
44B: True
44C: True
44D: False
44E: False
Closing volume (CV) is the lung volume below which alveoli begin to collapse. In healthy young adults, this volume is below the functional residual capacity (FRC); therefore, airway collapse does not occur during normal tidal breathing. However, in neonates and in adults above the age of about 40 years, CV is greater than the FRC and airway collapse occurs during normal breathing. Any cause of reduced FRC, such as supine positioning, general anaesthesia and the gravid uterus, can act in a similar fashion, with airway collapse occurring. CV can be measured by the single breath nitrogen wash out (Fowler's method). The point at which alveolar collapse begins is represented by an abrupt increase in the exhaled nitrogen concentration and corresponds to the CV.

Further reading

Hills GH. Respiratory physiology and anaesthesia. *Contin Educ Anaesth Crit Care Pain.* 2001; 1(2): 35–39.

45A: False
45B: True
45C: True
45D: True
45E: False

PONV is defined as retching, nausea or vomiting occurring within the first 24–48 h after surgery in inpatients. It is a well-recognized complication of general anaesthesia, occurring in 20–40% of patients, and up to 80% in those patients at high risk.

PONV is not only unpleasant; it can increase the duration of a hospital stay, increase readmissions to hospitals in outpatients, and rarely cause suture dehiscence, gastric aspiration and oesophageal rupture.

There are well-recognized factors that increase the risk of PONV. These can be considered as patient, anaesthetic and surgical factors.

Patient factors
- Female gender (three times more likely than male patients)
- Non-smokers (odds ratio of ~2)
- History of previous PONV
- History of motion sickness
- Age (for children risk increases with age over 3; adult risk decreases with age)

Anaesthetic factors
- Use of nitrous oxide (odds ratio 1.4)
- Volatile anaesthesia (increases risk four times)
- Intraoperative and postoperative opioids (dose-dependent)
- Duration of anaesthesia

Surgical factors
- Strabismus surgery in children
- Others, likely but no evidence in multivariate analysis
  - Gynaecological surgery
  - Ophthalmological surgery
  - Otological surgery
  - Emergency procedures
  - Gastrointestinal procedures
  - Postoperative pain
  - Ileus, gastric distension

Further reading

Pierre S, Whelan R. Nausea and vomiting after surgery. *Contin Educ Anaesth Crit Care Pain.* 2013; 13(1): 2–32.

46A: False
46B: False
46C: True
46D: True
46E: True

Iron is a mineral element that is an important component of haemoglobin, myoglobin and cytochromes. It is absorbed from the diet either as haem, from meat, or free iron. Iron absorption predominantly takes place in the duodenum and jejunum. Only 5–25% of ingested iron is absorbed; the rest is excreted in the faeces.

Iron is absorbed into the enterocyte by pinocytosis (haem iron) or by active transport (free iron). Within the enterocyte, haem iron is broken down into free iron. Free iron is stored as ferritin by binding with apoferritin. Much of this iron is lost as enterocytes are shed. Some of the free iron is transported across the basement membrane bound to an intracellular transport protein. Once released into the circulation, it binds to transferrin.

The amount absorbed depends on total body iron stores. In low iron states, upregulation of intestinal iron receptors and intracellular transport proteins can increase absorption.

Seventy percent of total body iron is incorporated as the central iron atom in the haem part of haemoglobin; 10% is incorporated in myoglobin, and 20% is stored as ferritin in cells.

Further reading

Hans G, Jones N. Preoperative anaemia. *Contin Educ Anaesth Crit Care Pain.* 2013; 13(3): 71–74.

Smith T, Pinnock C, Lin T. *Fundamentals of Anaesthesia.* 3rd ed. Cambridge: Cambridge University Press; 2009.

47A: True
47B: False
47C: True
47D: False
47E: False
Carbon dioxide (CO_2) is a product of cellular metabolism (200 ml·min^{-1} at rest) and is excreted via the lungs. Transport of carbon dioxide to the lungs occurs in the blood in three ways:

- Dissolved: 5% of carbon dioxide in arterial and 10% in venous blood. CO_2 is 20 times more soluble than oxygen and has a solubility coefficient of 0.231 mmol·litre^{-1}·kPa^{-1} at 37°C.
- Bound to proteins: predominantly haemoglobin. CO_2 rapidly combines with terminal uncharged amino groups to form carbamino compounds. In the case of haemoglobin, carbaminohaemoglobin compounds are effective hydrogen ion buffers. This is the method of transport of 6% of CO_2 in arterial blood and 30% in venous blood.
- As carbonic acid: this is the predominant mechanism of CO_2 transport, comprising 90% of CO_2 in arterial blood and 60% in venous blood. Red blood cell carbonic anhydrase catalyzes the reaction of carbon dioxide with water to form carbonic acid, which then freely dissociates to hydrogen ions and bicarbonate. Bicarbonate then diffuses out of the red blood cell in exchange for chloride ions, known as the Hamburger effect.

Further reading

Arthurs GJ, Sudhakar M. Carbon dioxide transport. *Contin Educ Anaesth Crit Care Pain.* 2005; 5(6): 207–210.

48A: True
48B: False
48C: False
48D: False
48E: True
Baroreceptors are stretch receptors located in the walls of the carotid sinus, aortic arch, atria, ventricles and pulmonary vessels.

Impulse generation is related to the degree of stretch, which in turn is related to blood pressure. Increased stretch increases discharge and vice versa. Discharge of impulses from the baroreceptors exert an inhibitory influence on the pressor centre in the rostral part of the ventral medulla, leading to vasodilatation and a reduction in heart rate. These effects lead to a fall in blood pressure.

Baroreceptors respond to both pressure and rate of change of pressure, and can respond to changes in arterial pressure, pulse pressure and heart rate. Atrial and ventricular baroreceptors also induce stimulation of the sino-atrial node leading to tachycardia (Bainbridge reflex).

Baroreceptors in the carotid sinus relay impulses to the central nervous system via the glossopharyngeal nerve, whereas aortic arch baroreceptors relay impulses via the vagus nerves.

Further reading

Foëx P, Sear JW. Hypertension: pathophysiology and treatment. *Contin Educ Anaesth Crit Care Pain.* 2004; 4(3): 71–75.

49A: True
49B: True
49C: False
49D: False
49E: True
Genetic defects affecting haemoglobin are the most common of all the genetic disorders. The defects either affect the production of the globin chains as in thalassaemias or the structure of the globin chain as in haemoglobinopathies.

The haemoglobin molecule in adults is usually made up of 2 α- and 2 β-globin chains. This gives the HbA form. HbA_2 is made up of 2 α- and 2 δ-chains but accounts for only 2.2–3.5% of the haemoglobin pool. Foetal haemoglobin (HbF) is composed of 2 α- and 2 γ-chains. At birth 50–95% of the infant's haemoglobin is of the foetal variety. These levels decline over the first 6 months to a point where only 1% of haemoglobin is HbF, which continues into adult life.

Further reading

Thomas, C, Lumb A. Physiology of haemoglobin. *Contin Educ Anaesth Crit Care Pain.* 2012; 12(5): 251–256.

50A: True
50B: False
50C: True
50D: True
50E: False

Gastrin is secreted by G cells in the stomach antrum and the duodenum. Secretion is stimulated by vagal stimulation, distension of the antrum and duodenum and by the ingestion of amino acids and peptides and alcohol and caffeine. Effects of gastrin are increased gastric acid production, secretion of pepsinogens and mucous. It also increases gastric motility and constricts the pyloric sphincter, reducing gastric emptying.

Somatostatin is released by D cells in the stomach; release is stimulated by gastric acidity.

Secretin is released by the S cells in the duodenum and jejunum; release is stimulated by increased acidity in duodenal chyme.

Cholecystokinin (CCK) is released by I cells in the duodenum and jejunum; release is stimulated by an increase in the fat content in duodenal chyme.

Further reading

Jollife DM. Practical gastric physiology. *Contin Educ Anaesth Crit Care Pain*. 2009; 9(6): 173–177.

51A: True
51B: False
51C: True
51D: True
51E: False

Peripheral nociceptor impulses travel in peripheral nerves whose cell bodies are located in the dorsal root ganglia in the spinal canal. The grey matter in the spinal cord is divided into 10 areas, known as Rexed laminae. Laminae I to VI make up the dorsal horn, VII to IX the ventral horn and X is located around the central canal.

Nociceptive information is transmitted from the dorsal horn to the thalamus and higher centres via the lateral and anterior spinothalamic tracts. There is also transmission through the spinoreticular and spinomesencephalic tract. These collectively make up the antero-lateral funiculus. The spinothalamic tract ascends a few segments and then decussates to the contralateral side through the ventral white commissure.

Further reading

Ellis H, Feldman S, Harrop-Griffiths W. *Anatomy for Anaesthetists*. 8th ed. Oxford: Wiley-Blackwell; 2003.

52A: True
52B: False
52C: True
52D: False
52E: True

The larynx is a cartilaginous structure and is composed of the thyroid, cricoid, two arytenoid, two corniculate and two cuneiform cartilages. It is also in approximation to the epiglottic cartilage.

The larynx has intrinsic and extrinsic muscles. All intrinsic muscles, except the cricothyroid, are innervated by the recurrent laryngeal nerve. Sensation to the larynx above the vocal cords comes from the internal laryngeal nerve and below the vocal cords from the recurrent laryngeal nerve. The vestibular folds are fixed folds on each side of the larynx lateral to the vocal folds. The cricothyroid muscle supplied by the external laryngeal nerve serves to tense the vocal cords. The thyroarytenoid relaxes the cords. The lateral cricoarytenoids adduct the cords whereas the posterior cricoarytenoids abduct them. The transverse arytenoid closes the posterior part of the rima glottidis.

Intrinsic Muscle	Function
Cricothyroid	Tenses vocal cords
Thyroarytenoid	Relaxes vocal cords
Lateral cricoarytenoids	Adduct cords
Posterior cricoarytenoids	Abduct cords
Transverse arytenoid	Closes posterior part of rima glottidis

Further reading

Snell RS. *Clinical Anatomy*. 7th ed. Philadelphia: Lippincott Williams & Wilkins; 2003.

53A: False
53B: False
53C: True
53D: False
53E: True

The word *dermatome* is derived from Greek and means 'skin slice'. A dermatome is an area of skin supplied by a single spinal nerve. There are 8 cervical nerves, 12 thoracic, 5 lumbar and 5 sacral; however, C1 has no dermatome.

The dermatomes along the thorax and abdomen are arranged like a stack. The pattern along the arms and legs is different, with the most distal portion of the limb being supplied by the middle dermatome of all those supplying the limb. Following is a list of the spinal nerves and characteristic anatomical points:

C2 Occipital protuberance
C3 Supraclavicular fossa
C4 Acromioclavicualr joint
C5 Radial side of antecubital fossa, proximal to elbow
C6 Thumb

C7	Middle finger
C8	Little finger
T1	Ulnar side of antecubital fossa, proximal to elbow
T2	Apex of axilla
T4	Horizontal level of nipple line
T10	Horizontal level of umbilicus
T12	Inguinal ligament
L4	Medial malleolus
L5	Middle toe
S1	Lateral aspect of calcaneus
S2	Midpoint of popliteal fossa
S3	Tuberosity of ischium
S4/5	Perianal region

Further reading

Whitaker RH, Borley NR. *Instant Anatomy*. 3rd ed. Oxford: Wiley-Blackwell; 2005.

54A: False
54B: False
54C: True
54D: False
54E: False

The anatomy of the spine is important in anaesthetic practice, particularly when performing central neuraxial blockade. The spine consists of 7 cervical vertebrae, 12 thoracic vertebrae, 5 lumbar vertebrae and the sacrum and coccyx. Each of the vertebrae is in contact with those above and below, and is connected to them via a number of joints and ligaments.

There are cartilaginous joints between vertebral bodies and synovial joints between the articular processes. The bodies between adjacent vertebrae are covered by a thin plate of hyaline cartilage. Sandwiched between these plates are intervertebral discs made of fibrocartilage. They make up one-fourth of the length of the vertebral column, and are thicker in the cervical and lumbar region.

Longitudinal ligaments run down the anterior and posterior surfaces of the vertebral column. The spines of the vertebrae are connected by the supraspinous and interspinous ligaments. The ligamentum flavum connects adjacent laminae.

The spinal cord begins superiorly at the foramen magnum as a continuation of the medulla oblongata. In adults, it usually terminates at the lower border of the first lumbar vertebrae. It then tapers below to form the conus medullaris. The filum terminale is a prolongation of pia mater that extends from the conus to the coccyx. The cauda equina (Latin: 'horse's tail') is composed of the roots of the lumbar and sacral nerves below the cord. At each level there are anterior and posterior nerve roots that pass through the subarachnoid space and unite as they leave the intervertebral foramina to form a spinal nerve that divides into an anterior ramus and a posterior ramus.

Further reading

Richardson J, Groen G. Applied epidural anatomy. *Contin Educ Anaesth Crit Care Pain*. 2005; 5(3): 98–100.

55A: False
55B: False
55C: True
55D: False
55E: True

Starvation is the complete absence of dietary intake. Glucose supplies to the brain are a priority and are provided by glycogenolysis and the release of glucose into the blood for the first 48 hours. After this time, gluconeogenesis is triggered by low insulin levels and high glucagon levels, which stimulate amino acid release. This is an inefficient system, yielding 1 gram of glucose for every 1.75 grams of protein catabolism, and there is a coexistent reduction in glucose requirements. Ketogenesis ensues after 3 days when very low levels of insulin trigger the release of fatty acids such as ketoacids, acetoacetate and β-hydroxybutyrate. These can be used directly as a fuel source by most tissues, including the brain. In starvation the level of ketones rises from the normal 0.2 to 0.6 mmol·L^{-1}. Death from starvation occurs after 60 days on average, when fat and protein stores have been depleted. Death usually results from respiratory failure and respiratory tract infection due to failed clearance of secretions.

Further reading

Denner AM, Townley SA. Anorexia nervosa: perioperative implications. *Contin Educ Anaesth Crit Care Pain*. 2009; 9(2): 61–64.

56A: False
56B: False
56C: True
56D: True
56E: True

The afferent limb of the vomiting reflex is activated by a range of stimuli, including those from the gastrointestinal (GI) tract, the chemoreceptor trigger zone and the vestibular system. Gastrointestinal tract afferents are carried in the vagus nerve, which supplies mechanoreceptors (which respond to gut distension) and chemoreceptors (which detect toxins and irritants within the lumen). The chemoreceptor trigger zone lies outwith the blood–brain barrier and has muscarinic, histaminic, dopaminergic (D_2), opioid (μ), serotenergic (5-HT$_3$) and alpha receptors.

Further reading

Pierre S, Whelan R. Nausea and vomiting after surgery. *Contin Educ Anaesth Crit Care Pain*. 2013; 13(1): 28–32.

57A: False
57B: True
57C: True
57D: False
57E: False

CSF is a specialized extracellular fluid, which bathes the central nervous system within the subarachnoid space and the ventricles. CSF is produced at a rate of 0.3 ml·min^{-1}; in total 500 ml·day^{-1}. The total volume of CSF is normally 120–150 ml, which is turned over four times per day. CSF is formed by active filtration of plasma. Compared with plasma, CSF contains less protein, bicarbonate, glucose, sodium and potassium but more chloride and a higher partial pressure of carbon dioxide.

Substance	Plasma	CSF
Protein	70 g/L	0.3 g/L
Bicarbonate	25 mmol/L	23 mmol/L
Glucose	8 mmol/L	4.8 mmol/L
Sodium	150 mmol/L	147 mmol/L
Potassium	4.6 mmol/L	2.9 mmol/L
Chloride	100 mmol/L	112 mmol/L
PCO$_2$	5.3 kPa	6.6 kPa

Further reading

Power I, Kam P. *Principles of Physiology for the Anaesthetist*. 2nd ed. London: Hodder Arnold; 2008.

Smith T, Pinnock C, Lin T. *Fundamentals of Anaesthesia*. 3rd ed. Cambridge: Cambridge University Press; 2009. p. 253–258.

58A: True
58B: True
58C: True
58D: True
58E: False

Ammonia is constantly produced in tissues; however, it is toxic to the central nervous system. Ammonia levels are kept low as it is released as glutamine or alanine, rather than free ammonia, and is rapidly removed from the blood by the liver. Sources of ammonia are amino acid metabolism, glutamine (in the nephron and intestine), urea (which is broken down in the gastrointestinal tract by bacteria), and the catabolism of purines and pyramidines. Beta-hydroxybutyrate is a ketone.

Further reading

Stewart MJ, Shepherd J, et al. *Clinical Biochemistry: An Illustrated Colour Text*. 4th ed. Edinburgh: Churchill Livingstone; 2011.

59A: False
59B: True
59C: False
59D: True
59E: True

The pancreas is a gland with both exocrine and endocrine functions, which regulate carbohydrate metabolism, digestion and serum glucose concentration. The pancreas is divided into lobules by connective tissue septae; each lobule contains an exocrine secretory unit, the acinus, which drains secretions into a ductile, then the pancreatic duct. Between the acini and the ducts are the islets of Langerhans, which have endocrine functions.

Approximately 1.5 litres of pancreatic fluid is produced each day, containing digestive enzymes and bicarbonate. The digestive enzymes are trypsinogen, chymotripsinogen, carboxypeptides, ribonuclease, deoxyribonuclease, lipase and amylase. These enzymes are responsible for the degradation of fats, carbohydrates and proteins in the small bowel. Bicarbonate is produced by the epithelial cells of the pancreatic ductules and acts to neutralize the gastric acid in the duodenum.

Further reading

Power I, Kam P. *Principles of Physiology for the Anaesthetist*. 2nd ed. London: Hodder Arnold; 2008.

Young S, Thompson JP. Severe acute pancreatitis. *Contin Educ Anaesth Crit Care Pain*. 2008; 8(4): 125–128.

60A: True
60B: False
60C: False
60D: True
60E: False

There are three main types of muscle fibres: types 1, 2 and 3.

Type 1 fibres are slow, oxidative fibres and are red in appearance. They are slow metabolically and mechanically and perform continuous slow contraction (e.g. the paraspinal muscles). Type 1 fibres have a high oxidative capacity and are able to sustain workloads for long periods; they have a high myoglobin content and do not tend to build up an oxygen debt. These fibres have an abundance of mitochondria, a good capillary blood supply and use predominantly aerobic metabolism of fatty acids.

Type 2 (also known as type 2B) fibres are fast, glycolytic fibres, which are white in colour. These fibres are fast metabolically and mechanically, capable of sustaining an intense workload for a short time only. Type 2 fibres depend on glycolysis predominantly for fuel metabolism and build up an oxygen debt. Type 2B fibres are found in oculomotor and small hand muscles and in sprinters' leg muscles.

Type 3 (also known as type 2A) fibres are fast oxidative fibres. These fibres have a fast contraction speed with high myosin ATPase activity and are red in colour.

They are progressively recruited when additional effort is required. They have a good capillary supply, plentiful mitochondria and myoglobin, and undergo aerobic metabolism of glucose and fatty acids for fuel.

Further reading

Hopkins, PM. Skeletal muscle physiology. *Contin Educ Anaesth Crit Care Pain.* 2006; 6(1): 1–6.

1. Sarin:
- A. Is a short-acting anticholinesterase agent
- B. Pharmacodynamic effects may be reversed by Pralidoxime
- C. Pharmacokinetic effects are reversed by Malathion
- D. Recovery of anticholinesterase activity occurs when sarin diffuses away from the synapse
- E. Is highly volatile

2. Lithium:
- A. Antagonizes antidiuretic hormone (ADH)
- B. Has a wide therapeutic window
- C. Potentiates the effects of neuromuscular blocking drugs
- D. Causes weight loss
- E. Increases serum calcium levels

3. The following are correct:
- A. Diastereoisomers are molecules that contain two dissimilar groups joined to carbon atoms linked by a double bond or ring structure
- B. Isoflurane and enflurane exhibit chain isomerism
- C. Dobutamine and dihydrocodeine exhibit dynamic geometric isomerism
- D. Butane is a chain isomer of isobutane
- E. Isoprenaline and methoxamine have the same molecular weight

4. The following pharmacokinetics statements are correct:
- A. In a three-compartment model, drugs move between the compartments in an exponential manner
- B. The time taken for the patient to wake at the end of an infusion is the context-sensitive half-life
- C. After five time constants, a drug given as an infusion will reach steady state
- D. A drug with a low volume of distribution is likely to be lipid soluble
- E. In a one-compartment model, the natural log of the function $C = C_0 e^{-kt}$ gives a straight line

5. **Ecstasy (MDMA) toxicity is associated with:**
   A. Rhabdomyolysis
   B. Panic disorders
   C. Cerebrovascular events
   D. Isolated acute renal failure
   E. Serotonin syndrome

6. **The following drugs have a site of action that is an enzyme:**
   A. Warfarin
   B. Atracurium
   C. Aspirin
   D. Neostigmine
   E. Erythromycin

7. **Desmopressin:**
   A. Has anticoagulant effects
   B. Is used in the management of major haemorrhage
   C. May cause acute coronary syndrome
   D. Commonly causes hypernatraemia
   E. Reduces plasma activity of coagulation factor VIII

8. **Aminophylline:**
   A. Is used in life-threatening asthma
   B. Is selective for the phosphodiesterase III enzyme
   C. Has a wide therapeutic window
   D. May cause arrhythmias
   E. Is a xanthine derivative

9. **The following pairings are correct:**
   A. Cisplatin: alkylating agent
   B. Methotrexate: anti-metabolite
   C. Bleomycin: topoisomerase enzyme
   D. Cyclophosphamide: interference with mitotic processes
   E. Paclitaxel: cross-linking of DNA

10. **The following drugs exist as racemic mixtures:**
    A. Isoflurane
    B. Bupivicaine
    C. Sevoflurane
    D. Propofol
    E. Atropine

11. **The following drugs are naturally occurring:**
    A. Hyoscine
    B. Phenylephrine
    C. Digoxin
    D. Heparin
    E. Ephedrine

12. The following drugs need to be protected from ultraviolet light:
A. Sodium nitroprusside
B. Noradrenaline
C. Diazepam
D. Glyceryl trinitrate
E. Ethylchloride

13. Atropine:
A. Is a quaternary amine
B. Is a non-competitive antagonist at the muscarinic acetylcholine receptor
C. Reduces atrioventricular conduction time
D. Increases physiological dead space
E. Does not cross the blood–brain barrier

14. Heparin:
A. Binds reversibly to antithrombin
B. Prolongs thrombin time
C. Prolongs bleeding time
D. Is only partially inhibited by protamine
E. Is used in the treatment of disseminated intravascular coagulation

15. The following drugs are not safe to use in porphyria:
A. Thiopental
B. Midazolam
C. Propofol
D. Atracurium
E. Diclofenac

16. Tramadol:
A. Has two isomers
B. Is an agonist at the κ-opioid receptor
C. Inhibits noradrenaline reuptake
D. Is predominantly excreted in the bile
E. Can be used to treat postoperative shivering

17. The following drugs do not have positive inotropic activity:
A. Digoxin
B. Glucagon
C. Noradrenaline
D. Hydrocortisone
E. Milrinone

18. Propofol:
A. Is almost entirely unionized at physiological pH
B. Has a brief duration of action due to rapid metabolism
C. Has a pKa of 7.6
D. 40% is excreted unchanged in the urine
E. Is 98% plasma protein-bound

19. Nitrous oxide:
  A. Is 20 times more water soluble than nitrogen
  B. Increases intracranial pressure
  C. Acts by inhibiting activity at the $GABA_A$ receptor
  D. Increases duration of induction with other volatile agents
  E. Can cause sub-acute combined degeneration of the cord

20. Pethidine:
  A. Is bound to α-1-acid glycoprotein in the circulation
  B. Is more lipid soluble than morphine
  C. Has pro-convulsant metabolites
  D. Does not accumulate in renal failure
  E. Can accumulate in the foetus

21. Measures to reduce heat loss through radiation in theatre include:
  A. Warm intravenous infusions
  B. Forced air warming blankets
  C. Ensure the theatre environment is warm
  D. Neuraxial blockade
  E. Humidification of dry inspired gases

22. The following are correct of mechanisms of filtration:
  A. The physical prevention of large particles from passing through pores of a filtration material is the process of inertial impaction
  B. Diffusional interception captures very small particles due to their Brownian motion
  C. Dust particles can be filtered through gravitational settling
  D. Smaller particles exhibit Brownian motion to a higher degree
  E. Electrostatic attraction occurs when small particles collide with the filtration medium due to inertia

23. The two photons released by a laser are:
  A. Monochromatic
  B. Coherent
  C. Of the same wavelength
  D. Parallel
  E. Of low energy intensity

24. Magnetic resonance imaging:
  A. Uses ionizing radiation to produce a three-dimensional image
  B. Uses liquid hydrogen to cool the superconducting magnet to absolute zero
  C. Has a magnetic field strength that is 100 times stronger than the earth's magnetic field
  D. Produces images of the body by the interaction between oxygen molecules in the body tissues and a superimposed magnetic field
  E. Uses a magnet that cannot be easily switched off

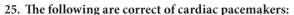

25. **The following are correct of cardiac pacemakers:**
    A. Electromagnetic interference is commonly from microwave or radiofrequency waves
    B. It is not safe to bring a mobile phone within 1 metre
    C. Modern pacemakers are monopolar
    D. Defibrillation can cause pacemaker resetting or damage
    E. Peripheral nerve stimulators can interfere with pacemaker function

26. **Anaesthetic gas scavenging:**
    A. Requires a low pressure vacuum system
    B. Should achieve minimum flows of 30 L·min^{-1}
    C. Is powered solely by patient's expiratory flow
    D. Uses the same piped medical vacuum as suction
    E. Uses 21 mm connectors

27. **The following statements are correct:**
    A. Pulse oximetry is inaccurate in neonates due to the presence of foetal haemoglobin
    B. The isobestic point for oxygenated and deoxygenated haemoglobin is 805 micrometres in the infrared spectrum
    C. Pulse oximetry has an accuracy of ±2% at an oxygen saturation range of 50–100%
    D. Beer's law states that the absorbance of light passing through a medium is proportional to the concentration of the medium
    E. The pulse oximeter will overestimate oxygen saturation in the presence of methaemoglobin

28. **The centralized vacuum system:**
    A. Generates a negative pressure of –40 kPa
    B. Accommodates an airflow rate of 53 L·min^{-1}
    C. Should have two vacuum outlets per operating theatre
    D. Should have two vacuum outlets per anaesthetic room
    E. Outlets are recognized by a yellow colour coding system

29. **Using distilled water, at a temperature of 22°C and under a pressure of 10 kPa, the flow through 110 cm tubing with an internal diameter of 4 mm is:**
    A. 40–80 ml·min^{-1} through a 20G cannula
    B. 130–220 ml·min^{-1} through a 16G cannula
    C. 75–120 ml·min^{-1} through a 20G cannula
    D. 250–360 ml·min^{-1} through a 20G cannula
    E. 250–360 ml·min^{-1} through a 14G cannula

30. **The following statements are correct:**
    A. The application of a voltage across an inductor will cause current to flow immediately
    B. The unit of inductance is the Becquerel (Bq)
    C. Inductors have low resistance to DC
    D. Inductors have high impedance to low-frequency AC signals
    E. Inductors have low impedance to low-frequency AC signals

31. Which of the following definitions are correct:
A. The first law of thermodynamics allows temperature to be defined
B. The zeroth law states that energy can neither be created nor destroyed; it can only be converted from one form to another
C. The cooling of an anaesthetized patient is explained by the second law of thermodynamics
D. The third law of thermodynamics states that the entropy of an object at absolute zero is zero
E. The fourth law of thermodynamics states that if two systems are in thermal equilibrium with a third system then they must be in equilibrium with each other

32. Oxygen analysis:
A. In theatre detection typically uses a paramagnetic cell
B. The paramagnetic analyzer works due to the atomic number of oxygen
C. Can be performed in the research setting using infrared absorption spectroscopy
D. Blood gas analysis utilizes the Severinghaus electrode
E. Using mass spectrometry is not widespread in theatres

33. The following pairings are correct:
A. Cylinder and NIST
B. Schrader valve and gas hosing
C. Pipeline gas and 4 bar pressure
D. Medical oxygen hose and black
E. Nitrous oxide cylinder and French blue

34. When using invasive blood pressure monitoring:
A. It cannot be used when blood flow is non-pulsatile
B. The systolic pressure will be higher than that measured by non-invasive blood pressure
C. The cannula used should be short and tapering
D. A constant infusion of saline at a rate of 2–4 ml·h⁻¹ is needed to keep the cannula patent
E. Raising the transducer 10 cm above the right atrium will reduce the blood pressure by 7.5 mmHg

35. Gas cylinders:
A. Have a plastic disc around the neck, which denotes what gas the cylinder contains
B. Have a NIST system on the valve block to prevent incorrect connection to the yoke of the anaesthetic machine
C. Containing Entonox™ must be stored in an area above 10°C
D. Containing oxygen has an absolute pressure of 137 bar
E. Containing carbon dioxide are grey

36. **When assessing neuromuscular blockade:**
    A. The TOF (Train of Four) Watch machine uses mechanomyography to assess neuromuscular block
    B. Electromyography is affected by diathermy
    C. Tetanic stimulation uses a frequency of 50–200 Hz
    D. Small degrees of residual block are more easily seen with TOF compared to double-burst stimulation
    E. It is important for a nerve stimulator to deliver a constant voltage

37. **The normal distribution:**
    A. Is also known as the Gaussian distribution
    B. Contains 95% of the data within ±2 standard deviations of the mean
    C. In its standard form has a mean of 0 and a standard deviation of 1
    D. Has the mode, median and mean equal in value
    E. Is positively skewed if the mean is larger in value than the mode

38. **Which of the following statements regarding data are correct:**
    A. Integer data is a subtype of interval data
    B. Categorical data are discrete
    C. Categorical data are quantitative
    D. Interval data is continuous
    E. Ordinal data can be pseudo-quantitative

39. **Regarding the colligative properties of solutions:**
    A. Increasing individual solute concentration has no effect on osmotic pressure
    B. Increasing solute concentration elevates the freezing point of a solvent
    C. Reduction of vapour pressure of a solvent in presence of a solute also elevates the boiling point
    D. Raoult's law relates molar concentration of a solute to depression of the freezing point
    E. Increase in vapour pressure of a solvent occurs proportionally to increase in molar concentration of the solute

40. **Regarding surface tension:**
    A. It exists at air–liquid interfaces
    B. When acting on a sphere results in greater pressure gradients the smaller the sphere
    C. It increases the surface tension within an alveolus, reducing the likelihood of collapse
    D. The pressure gradient acting within an alveolus is 8 multiplied by the surface tension divided by the radius
    E. Laplace's law states the pressure across the wall of a sphere is 4 multiplied by the surface tension divided by diameter

41. In calcium homeostasis:
A. Parathyroid hormone increases bone calcium resorption
B. Calcitonin is secreted by thyroid parafollicular cells
C. Parathyroid hormone is a glycopeptide secreted by chief cells of the parathyroid gland
D. Calcitonin increases renal calcium excretion
E. Ionized calcium acts indirectly to increase parathyroid hormone production

42. Considering bicarbonate:
A. Normal serum level is approximately 24 mmol·L^{-1}
B. It is responsible for 80% of carbon dioxide carriage in blood
C. 80% of filtered bicarbonate is reabsorbed by the kidney
D. It is reabsorbed in the distal convoluted tubule
E. Acidic urine occurs if plasma concentration is high

43. Functional residual capacity:
A. Is calculated by body plethysmography
B. Is equal to the sum of the residual volume and forced expiratory volume
C. Is the volume at which pulmonary vascular resistance is maximal
D. Is approximately 2500 ml in an adult male
E. Is not affected by gender

44. Hypoxic pulmonary vasoconstriction:
A. Is controlled by the central nervous system
B. Is reduced by volatile anaesthetic agents
C. Is inhibited by propofol
D. Is inhibited by vasodilators
E. Directs blood flow away from hypoxic regions of the lung

45. The following physiological changes may be seen in polycythaemia:
A. Increase in blood viscosity
B. Normal cardiac output
C. Reduction in total blood volume
D. Hypertension
E. Cyanosis

46. The effects on lungs of intermittent positive pressure ventilation include:
A. Increased right ventricular filling
B. Reduced surfactant production
C. Reduced V/Q mismatching
D. Increasing alveolar dead space
E. Alveolar recruitment

47. During pregnancy:
A. Carbon dioxide production decreases, resulting in reduced PaCO$_2$
B. Cardiac output increases due to increased contractility
C. Functional residual capacity is reduced by 20% at term
D. Oxygen consumption is increased by up to 60%
E. Plasma concentrations of all clotting factors increase

48. **The following physiological changes are seen with ageing:**
    A. Decreased stroke volume
    B. Increased lung compliance
    C. Increased cerebral blood flow
    D. Reduced residual volume
    E. Increased heart rate

49. **Non-respiratory functions of the lung include:**
    A. Removal of circulating histamine
    B. Inactivation of bradykinin
    C. Conversion of angiotensin II
    D. Removal of leukotrienes
    E. Removal of prostaglandin E2 and F2α

50. **Haemoglobin:**
    A. Is known as methaemoglobin when the ferrous ion is reduced to the ferric form
    B. Affinity for oxygen is reduced by an increase in pH, partial pressure of carbon dioxide, temperature and the concentration of 2,3-DPG
    C. Has 240 times the affinity for carbon monoxide than it has for oxygen
    D. Binding with hydrogen ions is greater in the deoxygenated form compared with the oxygenated form
    E. Is composed of an iron-porphyrin compound joined to four globin molecules

51. **Maternal pain during labour:**
    A. Is transmitted by C fibres only
    B. Is partially transmitted by somatic nerves during the first stage
    C. Is referred to the T10–S4 dermatomes during the first stage
    D. Is associated with decreased uteroplacental blood flow
    E. Nerves from the uterus, lower segment and cervix accompany the thoracolumbar and sacral sympathetic outflow

52. **With respect to the anatomy of the heart:**
    A. The base of the heart is composed only of the right and left ventricle
    B. The coronary sinus opens into the lower part of the right atrium
    C. There is a moderator band present in both ventricles
    D. The left atrium is normally larger than the right atrium
    E. The right coronary artery opens into the anterior aortic sinus

53. **Cerebrospinal fluid:**
    A. The total volume in an adult is 150 ml
    B. Is produced by the arachnoid granulations of the lateral, third and fourth ventricles
    C. Leaves the fourth ventricle via the median foramen of Monro
    D. Leaves the fourth ventricle via the lateral foramina of Lushka
    E. Pressure in the lateral decubitus position is 70 to 180 mmCSF in a normal adult

54. The following statements about the antecubital fossa are correct:
A. The borders are the pronator teres, brachioradialis, and a line between the medial and lateral epicondyles
B. The floor of the fossa is reinforced by the bicipital aponeurosis
C. The contents from medial to lateral are the median nerve, brachial artery, biceps tendon and radial nerve
D. The cephalic vein lies medially on the arm
E. The brachial artery is an end artery

55. Spinal cord hemisection will cause ipsilateral loss of:
A. Proprioception
B. Pain sensation
C. Temperature sensation
D. Fine touch sensation
E. Motor weakness

56. Functions of the lymphatic system include:
A. Drainage of interstitial fluid
B. Absorption of protein from gastrointestinal absorption
C. Absorption of molecules accrued in inflamed tissues
D. Returning protein from the interstitium to the circulation
E. Absorption of fat derived from gastrointestinal absorption

57. Cerebral blood flow:
A. Is 14% of the cardiac output at rest
B. Is 150 ml per 100 g brain tissue per min
C. Is constant over a MAP range of 80–180 mmHg
D. Increases linearly by 2–4% for every 0.13 kPa increase in $PaCO_2$
E. Increases linearly by 2–4% for every 0.13 kPa decrease in PaO_2

58. The following statements are correct:
A. pH is log_{10} of the hydrogen ion concentration
B. An acid is a substance that donates protons
C. The carbonic acid/bicarbonate buffer system is a closed system
D. At physiological pH, the hydrogen ion concentration is 40 mmol/L
E. The pKa of the carbonic acid/bicarbonate buffer system is 6.1

59. Tri-iodothyronine:
A. Is 10 times less potent than thyroxine
B. Is synthesized in the thyroid gland from the iodination of tryptophan molecules
C. Production is increased in the presence of thyroid stimulating hormone
D. Is predominantly transported in the plasma bound to albumin
E. Exerts its action by binding to intracellular receptors

60. During skeletal muscle contraction:

A. The M-line of the sarcomere shortens

B. Calcium binds the C subunit of troponin, causing a change in the I and T subunits

C. Actin forms cross-bridges with tropomyosin, shortening the sarcomere

D. Relaxation is a passive process

E. Stimulation of the ryanodine receptor causes calcium release from the sarcoplasmic reticulum

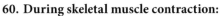

PAPER 4
ANSWERS

1A: False
1B: True
1C: False
1D: False
1E: True

Sarin is a highly potent, volatile, organophosphate agent used in chemical warfare. Organophosphate agents covalently bind to the esteratic site of the acetlylcholinesterase enzyme causing irreversible inhibition. Recovery of acetylcholinesterase activity occurs only when a new enzyme is synthesized.

Organophosphate poisoning results in profound overactivity of the parasympathetic nervous system with initial central excitation progressing to coma. A triphasic clinical syndrome occurs following exposure, consisting of an initial cholinergic phase (24–48 h), followed by an intermediate phase (4–18 days), with a subsequent delayed polyneuropathy phase (7–14 days after exposure). Patients are critically ill with bradycardia, bronchospasm, coma and convulsions, often necessitating critical care admission and ventilation.

Treatment of organophosphate poisoning involves atropine, anticonvulsants and oximes. Atropine is given in boluses or as an infusion until the full antimuscarinic effect has been achieved (pulse >90, dilated pupils, red dry skin). Atropine has no effect on the muscular symptoms as these are mediated by the nictonic receptors. Oximes (e.g. pralidoxime) act by reactivating acetylcholinesterase, detoxifying the unbound organophosphate agent through an endogenous anticholinergic effect.

Malathion is also an organophosphate compound with low toxicity in humans. It is used as a treatment for lice and scabies. It has no effect on the pharmacokinetics of sarin.

Further reading

Priya Nair V, Hunter JM. Anticholinesterases and anticholinergic drugs. *Contin Educ Anaesth Crit Care Pain.* 2004; 4(5): 164–168.

2A: True
2B: False
2C: True
2D: False
2E: True

Lithium is used as a mood stabilizer in the treatment of bipolar affective disorder and mania. Although the precise mechanism of action is unclear, it is believed that lithium acts by reducing neurotransmitter release in excitable cells by imitating the action of sodium ions.

Effects of lithium include seizures (with lowered seizure threshold in epileptics), increased muscle tone, ADH antagonism (causing polyuria and polydipsia), hypernatraemia, hypermagnasaemia, hypercalcaemia, prolongation of neuromuscular blockade and reducing the minimum alveolar concentration (MAC) of volatile anaesthetics. Side effects may include weight gain, hypothyroidism and tremor.

Lithium has a narrow therapeutic window with a therapeutic plasma concentration of 0.5 to 1.5 mmol·L^{-1}. Lithium toxicity causes vomiting, abdominal pain, ataxia, convulsions, arrhythmias and death. Lithium has 100% oral bioavailability and is not bound to plasma proteins. Lithium is excreted in the urine (95%) and sweat (5%).

Further reading

Flood A, Bodenham S. Lithium: mimicry, mania and muscle relaxants. *Contin Educ Anaesth Crit Care Pain.* 2010; 10(3): 77–80.

3A: False
3B: False
3C: False
3D: True
3E: True

Isomerism is the phenomenon whereby two chemical compounds have the same molecular composition (hence molecular weight) but differing structural arrangement. This results in differing physical or chemical properties. Isomerism may be structural (static or dynamic) or stereo (geometric or optical).

Structural isomerism: Two compounds have the same chemical formulae; however, the order of atomic bonds differs. Structural isomerism may be static or dynamic.

- Static isomerism: sub-classified into chain or position isomerism
    - Chain isomerism: the carbon skeleton of the molecule varies in structure; however, the position of the functional group is static (e.g. butane and isobutane)
    - Position isomerism: the carbon skeleton of the molecule is the same but the position of the functional group varies (e.g. isoflurane and enflurane)
- Dynamic isomerism: variant of structural isomerism where the molecule exists in differing molecular structure (keto or enol) depending on its environment (e.g. the structure of thiopentone tautomerizes depending on the environmental pH)

Other examples of structural isomers are dobutamine and dihydrocodeine; isoprenaline and methoxamine; prednisolone and aldosterone.

Stereoisomerism: two molecules of the same chemical or molecular formula differ in their 3-dimensional spatial arrangements. This may be geometric or optical.

- Geometric isomerism: a molecule with two dissimilar groups joined to two carbon atoms, which are linked by either a double bond or ring structure. If the groups are on the same side of the bond it is termed cis- and if they are on opposite sides, it is termed trans- (e.g. atracurium has 10 geometric stereoisomers).
- Optical stereosomerism: the molecule possesses a chiral atom (tetravalent atom, carbon or quaternary nitrogen, bound to four dissimilar groups) permitting the existence of two molecules, which are 'mirror images' of each other in three-dimensional view. These molecules cannot be superimposed on each other and are classified according to direction of rotation of polarized light (right/dextro-, or left/levo-rotatory) or in ascending order of molecular arrangement (right or left handed).
- Diastereoisomers are molecules containing more than one chiral centre.

Further reading

Calvey TN. Isomerism and anaesthetic drugs. *Acta Anaesthesiol Scand Suppl.* 1995; 106: 83–90.

E-learning Anaesthesia, Stocker, M. 07c_01_05 Isomers. [Online] Available from: http://portal.e-lfh.org.uk [Accessed 09 July 2012].

4A: True
4B: False
4C: False
4D: False
4E: True

Exponential processes occur at a rate proportional to the concentration gradient. As the process continues, the concentration gradient falls and the rate of the process will fall. The elimination of a drug from the plasma is an exponential process.

The exponential decay curve (of drug concentration against time) has the mathematical function:

$$y = e^{-x}$$

An exponential function can be described by its time constant and half-life.

Time constant

- Time taken for a process to be complete if the process had continued at its initial rate
- Corresponds with a reduction to 37% of the initial value
- A process is complete after three time constants

Half-life

- Time taken for the plasma concentration to reduce to 50% of its initial value
- A process is considered complete after five half-lives

Pharmacological compartment models divide the body into hypothetical compartments according to its size, affinity for the drug and blood flow. The simplest model is the one-compartment model, where a drug enters and is eliminated from one compartment only. The elimination of the drug from the one-compartment model is an exponential process, with the function $y = e^{-x}$ or $C = C_0 e^{-kt}$. Calculating the natural log (ln) of the function $C = C_0 e^{-kt}$ gives a straight-line graph with the gradient: $-k$. ($\ln C = \ln C_0 + \ln e^{-kt} = \ln C_0 - kt$).

A three-compartment model is more reflective of what happens *in vivo*, where the drug moves between the compartments, along its concentration gradient until equilibrium is established. The drug enters and leaves the body only from the first compartment. The movement of the drug between the compartments is exponential.

When a drug given as a constant infusion is stopped, the plasma concentration of the drug will behave according to the three-compartment model. The drug will be eliminated from the first compartment (plasma); however, redistribution from the second and third compartments will maintain the plasma drug concentration. The context-sensitive half-time is the time taken for the plasma concentration to fall by 50% at the end of an infusion. The context is the length of the infusion.

Further reading

Hill SA. Pharmacokinetics of drug infusions. *Contin Educ Anaesth Crit Care Pain.* 2004; 4(3): 76–80.

Roberts F, Freshwater-Turner D. Pharmacokinetics and anaesthesia. *Contin Educ Anaesth Crit Care Pain.* 2007; 7(1): 25–29.

5A: True
5B: True
5C: True
5D: False
5E: True

Ecstasy is an amphetamine-based drug. Its full name is 3,4-methylenedioxymeth-amphetamine, or MDMA (also known as 'the love drug', 'Adam' or 'E'). Ecstasy is associated with a number of minor symptoms including trismus, tachycardia and bruxism (nocturnal grinding of teeth). There is a hangover type effect that can last up to 5 days. More severe side effects include sudden death, hyperpyrexia, rhabdomyolysis, serotonin syndrome, isolated liver failure, panic attacks and hyponatraemia leading to cerebral oedema.

Ecstasy causes the release of the neurotransmitters 5-HT, dopamine and noradrenaline. It also prevents their reuptake, particularly 5-HT, leading to the serotonin syndrome. It then leads to depletion of serotonin stores over the next few days, which probably contributes to the typical midweek 'lows' experienced after recreational use on the weekends.

Isolated liver failure has been reported, rather than isolated renal failure, although multi-organ failure can occur. In addition, ecstasy is associated with cerebrovascular events in young people.

Further reading

Hall AP, Henry JA. Acute toxic effects of 'Ecstasy' (MDMA) and related compounds: overview of pathophysiology and clinical management. *Br J Anaesth*. 2006; 96(6): 678–685.

6A: True
6B: False
6C:True
6D: True
6E: False
Warfarin is a coumarin that acts by inhibiting the vitamin K epoxide reductase enzyme. The enzyme recycles oxidized vitamin K to its reduced form after it has carboxylated serum coagulation factors.

Atracurium is a non-depolarizing neuromuscular blocker of the benzylisoquinolinium class. It acts by blocking the nicotinic acetylcholine receptor at the neuromuscular junction. Atracurium acts as a reversible competitive inhibitor.

Aspirin acts on the cyclo-oxygenase (COX) enzymes. It has greater affinity for the *COX-1* enzyme compared to the *COX-2* enzyme. It irreversibly inhibits the enzymes preventing the synthesis of prostaglandin and thomboxanes from arachidonic acid.

Neostigmine binds to the anionic site of cholinesterase. This is the enzyme that breaks down acetylcholine in the neuromuscular junction.

Erythromycin acts by binding to the 50S subunit of the bacterial ribosome, interfering with aminoacyl translocation.

Further reading

Peck TE, Hill SA, Williams M. *Pharmacology for Anaesthesia and Intensive Care*. 3rd ed. Cambridge: Cambridge University Press; 2008.

7A: False
7B: False
7C: True
7D: False
7E: False
Desmopressin (1-desamino-8-D-arginine vasopressin, or DDAVP) is a synthetic analogue of antidiuretic hormone. DDAVP has procoagulant properties by promoting the release of von Willebrand's factor from the endothelium, increasing the activity of coagulation factor VIII and increasing the expression of platelet surface glycoprotein receptors to promote platelet adhesion. DDAVP is used therapeutically for its procoagulant effects in the management of haemophilia A (hereditary deficiency of coagulation factor VIII), and shortens bleeding time in patients with coagulopathy due to hepatic failure, uraemia or administration of NSAIDs. However, DDAVP is not used routinely in the management of major

haemorrhage due to the occurrence of side effects. These side effects are largely attributable to the antidiuretic effects, leading to water retention and dilutional hyponatraemia. DDAVP has little effect on systemic blood pressure; however, it may cause acute coronary syndrome in patients with coronary artery disease.

Further reading

Lethagen S. Desmopressin—a haemostatic drug: state-of-the-art review. *Eur J Anaesthesiol*. 1997; 14(Suppl): 1–9.

Ridley S, Taylor B, Gunning K. Medical management of bleeding in critically ill patients. *Contin Educ Anaesth Crit Care Pain*. 2007; 7(4): 116–121.

8A: True
8B: False
8C: False
8D: True
8E: True

Aminophylline is a methylated xanthine derivative that is used in the management of asthma, COPD and cardiac failure. It acts by inhibiting phosphodiesterase enzymes, preventing the breakdown of intracellular cyclic AMP (cAMP). The accumulation of cAMP causes a variety of tissue specific effects. There are a number of different phosphodiesterase enzymes; phosphodiesterase III (PDE III) is found in the cardiac myocyte and is specifically inhibited by drugs such as milrinone and enoximone. Aminophylline however is non-specific.

Aminophylline is a potent bronchodilator, increases the sensitivity of the respiratory centre to CO_2 and promotes contractility of the diaphragm. Cardiovascular effects are mild positive inotropy and chronotropy, reduced systemic blood pressure and arrhythmias. Other side effects of aminophylline are seizures, increased gastric acid production, diuresis and hypokalaemia.

Aminophylline has a narrow therapeutic window and rapid saturation of metabolizing cytochrome P450 enzymes occurs at higher doses. For this reason, aminophylline levels should be closely monitored and caution taken to avoid administration of interacting drugs such as erythromycin.

Further reading

Feneck R. Phosphodiesterase inhibitors and the cardiovascular system. *Contin Educ Anaesth Crit Care Pain*. 2007; 7(6): 203–207.

Stanley D, Tunnicliffe W. Management of life-threatening asthma in adults. *Contin Educ Anaesth Crit Care Pain*. 2008; 8(3): 95–99.

9A: True
9B: True
9C: True
9D: False
9E: False

The anaesthetist is likely to come across patients who are receiving chemotherapy. Patients undergoing chemotherapy treatment may need to undergo a number of cancer-related elective operations. There is also the likelihood of incidental emergency operations. Consequently, the anaesthetist should be aware of the types of chemotherapeutic agents and their associated complications. The common agents are alkylating agents, which cause cross-linking of DNA (cyclophosphamide, cisplatin); anti-metabolites (methotrexate, 5-fluorouracil); topoisomerase interactive agents (doxorubicin, bleomycin); and anti-microtubule agents, which interrupt mitotic and non-mitotic cellular processes (paclitaxel).

Further reading

Allan N, Siller C, Breen A. Anaesthetic implications of chemotherapy. *Contin Educ Anaesth Crit Care Pain*. 2012; 12(2): 52–56.

10A: True
10B: True
10C: False
10D: False
10E: True
Stereoisomerism is the existence of molecules with the same chemical constituents but different spatial arrangements. Geometric and optical are two forms of stereoisomerism. In optical stereoisomerism a chiral centre exists. This is either a carbon atom or a quaternary nitrogen atom. They have four bonds, with a different chemical group connected to each. This allows different arrangements of the chemical groups to the chiral centre. This produces molecules that are mirror images of each other and cannot be superimposed on each other. These mirror images are termed enantiomers. When prepared pharmaceutically, mixtures of these enantiomers are produced in equal proportions. This is termed a racemic mixture. Examples of drugs that are produced as racemic mixtures are the volatile anaesthetics (except sevoflurane), bupivacaine and atropine. Propofol and sevoflurane do not contain a chiral centre so have no enantiomers.

Further reading

Calvey TN. Isomerism and anaesthetic drugs *Acta Anaesthesiol Scand*. 1995; 106(Suppl): 83–90.

E-learning Anaesthesia, Stocker, M. 07c_01_05 Isomers. [Online] Available from: http://portal.e-lfh.org.uk.

11A: True
11B: False
11C: True
11D: True
11E: True
Hyoscine, also known as scopolamine, is an alkaloid drug that has muscarinic antagonist effects. It is extracted from the nightshade family of plants.

Scopolamine is named after the plant genus *Scopolia*. Hyoscine is from the scientific name for henbane, *Hyoscyamus niger*. Phenylephrine is a synthetic sympathomimetic. Digoxin is derived from the foxglove plant, *Digitalis*, and is a purified cardiac glycoside. Heparin is found naturally in the liver (hence the name) and in mast cell granules. It is a glycosaminoglycan and is used therapeutically as an anticoagulant. Its physiological role is less clear as anticoagulation is achieved mostly through heparin sulphate derived from endothelial cells. Ephedrine is a naturally occurring sympathomimetic. It is an alkaloid derived from the plants of the genus *Ephedra*. The plant grows on shores or on sandy soils, and the common name is Joint-pine or Brigham tea.

Further reading

Peck TE, Hill SA, Williams M. *Pharmacology for Anaesthesia and Intensive Care.* 3rd ed. Cambridge: Cambridge University Press; 2009.

12A: True
12B: True
12C: True
12D: False
12E: False
Ultraviolet (UV) light can cause oxidation, hydrolysis and loss of potency of some medications. These medications therefore need to be protected from UV light, are presented in amber ampoules and should be drawn up in amber syringes for administration, particularly if given as an infusion. The syringes can also be protected by wrapping in foil. Diazepam is presented as a solution in an amber ampoule but is usually administered as a bolus. Sodium nitroprusside and noradrenaline should be drawn up in an amber syringe as UV light can cause degradation, particularly with sodium nitroprusside. Glyceryl trinitrate and ethyl chloride are not affected by UV light.

Further reading

Peck TE, Hill SA, Williams M. *Pharmacology for Anaesthesia and Intensive Care.* 3rd ed. Cambridge: Cambridge University Press; 2009.

13A: False
13B: False
13C: True
13D: True
13E: False
Atropine is a naturally occurring alkaloid found in *Atropa belladonna* (or deadly nightshade). It is commercially available as a racemic mixture of *L*- and *D*-isomers, as tablets or clear colourless solution for injection.

It is an anticholinergic that competitively antagonizes acetylcholine at muscarinic receptors. It is readily absorbed from the gastrointestinal tract and has an oral bioavailability of up to 25%. Its tertiary amine structure allows it to cross

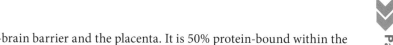
both the blood–brain barrier and the placenta. It is 50% protein-bound within the plasma and has a volume of distribution of 2–4 L·kg^{-1}.

Atropine is hydrolyzed in the liver and tissues and 94% is excreted in the urine.

It produces a tachycardia (occasionally preceded by an initial bradycardia) and increases cardiac output. It decreases atrioventricular conduction time and consequently can cause dysrhythmias. It causes bronchodilation and reduces bronchial as well as gastric, salivary and sweat gland secretions.

It can cause central anticholinergic syndrome and also has antiemetic effects and increases basal metabolic rate.

Further reading

Smith S, Scarth E, Sasada M. *Drugs in Anaesthesia and Intensive Care*. 4th ed. Oxford: Oxford University Press; 2011. p. 36–37.

14A: True
14B: True
14C: False
14D: False
14E: True

Unfractionated heparin is a naturally occurring anticoagulant extracted from bovine lung or porcine intestinal mucosa. It is used in the prevention and treatment of venous thromboembolism, disseminated intravascular coagulation and acute coronary syndromes.

Heparin acts by reversibly binding to circulating antithrombin III, and the resulting complex has enhanced ability to inhibit activated clotting factors XIII, XII, XI, X, IX, plasmin and thrombin.

It is administered intravenously or subcutaneously, and leads to prolongation of the thrombin time, whole blood clotting time and activated partial thromboplastin time (APTT). It does not affect the bleeding time. At least 4 hours should be left between discontinuation of heparin infusion and neuroaxial anaesthesia.

In addition, heparin inhibits platelet aggregation and leads to an increase in plasma-free fatty acids. It is metabolized in the kidneys, liver and reticuloendothelial system. Heparin-induced thrombocytopenia (HIT) occurs in 5% of patients on heparin infusions.

Heparin is specifically antagonized by protamine. This is a strong basic compound that binds with acidic heparin to form an inactive compound. One milligram of protamine will neutralize 100 IU of heparin.

Further reading

Barker R, Marval P. Venous thromboembolism: risks and prevention. *Contin Educ Anaesth Crit Care Pain*. 2011; 11(1): 18–23.

Peck TE, Hill SA, Williams M. *Pharmacology for Anaesthesia and Intensive Care*. 3rd ed. Cambridge: Cambridge University Press; 2008. Chapter 23, p. 335–337.

Smith S, Scarth E, Sasada M. *Drugs in Anaesthesia and Intensive Care*. 4th ed. Oxford: Oxford University Press; 2011. p. 166–167.

15A: True
15B: True
15C: False
15D: False
15E: True

Porphyrins are cyclical organic structures; the most important in humans is haem, the iron-containing constituents of haemoglobin, myoglobin, cytochromes and catalases.

Porphyria describes excessive production of porphyrin and porphyrin precursors seen in a group of diseases caused by acquired and genetic errors of metabolism. They are extremely rare in the UK population (1–2 per 100 000), the most common being acute intermittent porphyria (AIP), but high levels of porphyrins can lead to neurotoxicity in susceptible patients and neurovisceral crises.

The most relevant to anaesthetists are the acute porphyrias. These variants affect the enzymatic pathway of haem production in the liver and the cytochrome P450 system. Precipitating factors increase demand for haem in the liver and therefore increase flux through the haem pathway, leading to accumulation of substrates for the defective intermediary enzymes. In acute porphyrias, levels of 5-aminolaevulinic acid (5-ALA) are increased and, in some variants, elevated levels of porphobilogen can be used to detect acute crises.

Symptoms and signs of acute crises are thought to be due to neurological dysfunction in motor, sensory and autonomic nerves and the central nervous system, either due to a direct neurotoxic effect of 5-ALA, or due to haem deficiency.

General precipitants are often seen around the peri-operative period and include starvation, stress, dehydration and infection, but a large number of drugs are implicated in triggering acute crises.

Drugs known to be unsafe in acute porphyria include benzodiazepines, barbiturates and sevoflurane. Propofol, other inhalational anaesthetic agents and most non-depolarizing muscle relaxants are thought to be safe. Most opioid analgesics, with the exception of oxycodone, are thought to be safe but diclofenac is a known trigger.

Further reading

Findley H, Philips A, Cole D, Nair A. Porphyrias: implications for anaesthesia, critical care and pain medicine. *Contin Educ Anaes Crit Care Pain*. 2012; 12(3): 128–133.

16A: True
16B: True
16C: True
16D: False
16E: True

Tramadol is a synthetic opioid used in moderate-to-severe pain for its analgesic properties and is equipotent to pethidine in this respect.

It is presented as a racemic mixture of two enantiomers and is available both in tablet form and as a clear colourless solution for intramuscular or intravenous injection. It has good oral bioavailability of 68–100% and therefore the dose of 50–100 mg four times daily is the same regardless of route of administration. In children, the dose is 1–2 mg·kg⁻¹, 4–6 hourly.

Tramadol exhibits agonist activity at μ-, κ-and δ-opioid receptors but has a higher affinity for μ-opioid receptors. Tramadol also inhibits neuronal noradrenaline reuptake and enhances serotonin release, which may enhance its analgesic properties. It does not cause respiratory depression at therapeutic doses, and also causes less constipation than other opioids.

Tramadol is excreted mainly (90%) in the urine and its use should be avoided in patients with significant renal impairment. The dosage interval should be increased to 12-hourly in patients with renal or hepatic impairment as 85% is metabolized in the liver.

Further reading

Smith S, Scarth E, Sasada M. *Drugs in Anaesthesia and Intensive Care*. 4th ed. Oxford: Oxford University Press; 2011. p. 370–371.

17A: False
17B: False
17C: True
17D: False
17E: False

The term 'inotropy' refers to myocardial contractility. Positive inotropes act to increase myocardial contractility, usually via a common pathway resulting in increased calcium release into the myocyte, leading to increased actin-myosin cross-bridge formation and increased myocyte contractility. Stimulation of G-protein-coupled β-adrenoreceptors on cardiac muscle increases production of intracellular cyclic adenosine monophosphate (cAMP) and ultimately increases intracellular calcium. Phosphodiesterase inhibitors such as milrinone prevent the breakdown of cAMP by phosphodiesterases; the resulting increase in cAMP increasing intracellular calcium via protein kinase activation. Steroids such as hydrocortisone increase both number and activity of adrenoreceptors and therefore increase opportunity for β-adrenoreceptor activation. Glucagon similarly exerts its positive inotropic effect via this route. Digoxin again increases intracellular calcium but exerts its action by displacement of bound intracellular calcium due to increases in sodium ion concentration within the myocyte.

Further reading

Hasenfuss G, Teerlink JR. Cardiac inotropes: current agents and future directions. *Eur Heart J*. 2011; 32(15): 1838–1845.

Peck TE, Hill SA, Williams M. *Pharmacology for Anaesthesia and Intensive Care*. 3rd ed. Cambridge: Cambridge University Press; 2008. Chapter 12, p. 197–215.

18A: True
18B: False
18C: False
18D: False
18E: True

Propofol is an alkylated phenol derivative, 2,6-diisopropylphenol, used predominantly as an intravenous anaesthetic agent. It is a weak organic acid with a pKa of 11 and is therefore almost entirely unionized at physiological pH. It is 98% plasma protein-bound and has a volume of distribution of 4 L·kg⁻¹. Propofol is highly lipid soluble and is not water soluble. It is therefore presented as an oil-in-water emulsion containing 1 or 2% propofol, soya bean oil and purified egg phosphatide. These pharmacokinetic properties lead to rapid redistribution from the plasma into lipid-rich tissues and a brief duration of action after bolus administration, with a redistribution half-life of 1.3–4.1 minutes. This distribution follows a three-compartment pharmacokinetic model. Propofol is metabolized rapidly by glucuronide conjugation (40%) in the liver or to a quinol (60%), which is later hydroxylated and conjugated for excretion in the urine. Less than 1% is excreted unchanged.

Further reading

Schüttler J, Ihmsen H. Population pharmacokinetics of propofol: a multicenter study. *Anesthesiology*. 2000; 92(3): 727–738.

19A: False
19B: True
19C: False
19D: False
19E: True

Nitrous oxide (N₂O) is an inorganic compound used as an adjuvant to volatile agents in general anaesthesia as well as in combination with 50% oxygen for its analgesic properties as Entonox™. It is sweet smelling and has a minimum alveolar concentration of 105%, limiting its use as a sole agent for general anaesthesia. Despite its low solubility (blood:gas partition coefficient: 0.47), large amounts of nitrous oxide are absorbed into the pulmonary capillaries very rapidly when used at high concentrations. This is thought to be due to the disproportionately rapid rise in alveolar concentration seen when nitrous oxide is used in high concentrations (concentration effect), leading to a large concentration gradient between the alveolar gas and the capillary blood.

As a result of this concentration effect, concurrently administered volatile agents will also be concentrated within the alveolus, increasing their uptake due to an enhanced concentration gradient. This is known as the 'second gas effect', and is due to the rapid uptake of nitrous oxide from the alveolus, faster than nitrogen from the capillaries can move back into the alveolus in exchange. At the end of anaesthesia the reverse process occurs, resulting in large amounts of nitrous oxide diluting the oxygen within the alveolus, leading to a hypoxic concentration within the alveolus. This is known as diffusion hypoxia, or the Fink effect, and is avoided by administering supplementary oxygen.

Nitrous oxide is thought to act by non-competitive inhibition at excitatory NMDA receptors but has minimal effect at inhibitory $GABA_A$ receptors. It has beneficial analgesic properties, thought to be mediated within the periaqueductal grey matter and the locus ceruleus of the central nervous system. It increases both cerebral metabolic requirement for oxygen and cerebral blood flow and consequently increases intracranial pressure. As nitrous oxide is 30–35 times more soluble than nitrogen it can result in rapid expansion of air-filled spaces and should therefore be avoided in the presence of pneumothorax, bowel obstruction, middle ear surgery and intraocular gas. Its relationship with postoperative nausea and vomiting is thought to be due in part to changes in middle ear pressure and bowel distension as a result of this phenomenon. Prolonged administration of nitrous oxide (over 6 hours) has been shown to inhibit methionine synthetase by oxidation of the cobalamin (vitamin B_{12} form) of cobalt, interfering with DNA synthesis, particularly in the presence of vitamin B_{12} deficiency. It has been implicated in sub-acute combined degeneration of the cord. Nitrous oxide has been shown to be teratogenic in animal models, particularly in early pregnancy, and should therefore be avoided within the first trimester of pregnancy.

Further reading

Banks A, Hardman JG. Nitrous oxide. *Contin Educ Anaesth Crit Care Pain.* 2005; 5(5): 145–148.

20A: True
20B: True
20C: True
20D: False
20E: True

Pethidine is a synthetic, weakly basic, phenylpiperidine derivative, which acts at μ- and κ- (this may account for its anti-shivering effects) opioid receptors as well as having anticholinergic activity. It is highly lipid soluble (28 times more lipid soluble than morphine), and consequently has a more rapid onset of action than morphine but shares many of its opioid properties. It is one-tenth as potent, however, than morphine. Pethidine is commonly used for analgesia during labour, although its high lipid solubility results in significant placental transfer. It may also cause increases in amplitude of uterine contractions and, as a weak base, can become trapped in the acidic environment of the foetal circulation, where it can cause respiratory depression.

Pethidine may be administered via the oral, intramuscular or intravenous routes. It undergoes hepatic metabolism to pethidinic acid and norpethidine, which can accumulate significantly in renal failure due to its increased elimination half-life. Norpethidine is an active metabolite half as potent as pethidine and can cause seizures if it accumulates, as it has pro-convulsant properties and may therefore be contraindicated in severe pregnancy-induced hypertension.

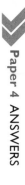

Further reading

Fortescue C, Wee MYK. Analgesia in labour: non-regional techniques. *Contin Educ Anaesth Crit Care Pain.* 2005; 5(1): 9–13.

Smith S, Scarth E, Sasada M. *Drugs in Anaesthesia and Intensive Care.* 4th ed. Oxford: Oxford University Press; 2011. p. 276–277.

21A: True
21B: True
21C: True
21D: False
21E: False
Heat loss in theatre occurs through five main mechanisms: radiation, convection, evaporation, respiration and conduction.

Radiation

Accounts for approximately 40% of heat loss. Heat energy is transferred from hotter to cooler objects. This is more pronounced with a larger temperature gradient (e.g. vasodilation with GA or neuraxial blockade, cool operating theatre). Mechanisms to prevent heat loss through radiation include warm intravenous infusions, increasing ambient temperature and the use of space blankets and forced air warmers.

Convection

Accounts for about 30% of heat loss. Air adjacent to the body warms, causing the density of this air to reduce and rise away from the patient, forming convection currents. The result is continual loss of heat from the patient. Heat loss through convection is more pronounced in operating theatres with laminar flow and can be prevented by using forced air warmers.

Evaporation

Accounts for about 15% of heat loss. Evaporation of water on the body surface causes loss of latent heat. This occurs especially with large open wounds, such as in open abdominal, orthopaedic, burns and plastic reconstructive surgery. Evaporative losses can be reduced with laparoscopic surgery, the use of drapes and plastic coverings.

Respiration

Accounts for approximately 10% of heat loss. Heat loss through the respiratory tract occurs due to humidification of dry inspired gases and warming of cool inspired gases. This can be reduced using humidification devices.

Conduction

Accounts for only about 5% heat loss, where direct patient contact with cooler substances (e.g. metal operating table/drip stands) causes heat loss.

Further reading

Sullivan G, Edmondson C. Heat and temperature. *Contin Educ Anaesth Crit Care Pain*. 2008; 8(3): 104–107.

22A: False
22B: True
22C: True
22D: True
22E: False

Filtration devices act through five main mechanisms:

- Direct interception: physical prevention of large particles from passing through the small pores of the filtration medium (e.g. dust, large bacteria)
- Inertial impaction: small particles collide with the filtration medium due to inertial forces causing the particles to move in straight lines (due to intermolecular Van der Waals forces)
- Diffusional interception: very small particles move at high velocity in Brownian motion, increasing their effective cross-sectional area and increasing the likelihood of collision with the filtration medium
- Electrostatic attraction: the particles in the fibres of the filtration medium exert an electrostatic attraction to oppositely charged microbial particles
- Gravitational settling: large particles are subject to gravitational forces, which cause the particles to settle on the filtration medium rather than follow the stream of the gas flow

Further reading

Al Shaikh B, Stacey S. *Essentials of Anaesthetic Equipment*. 3rd ed. Philadelphia: Elsevier Health Sciences; 2007.

Wilkes AR. Breathing system filters. *Contin Educ Anaesth Crit Care Pain*. 2002; 2(5): 151–154.

23A: True
23B: True
23C: True
23D: True
23E: False

LASER is an acronym, standing for Light Amplification by Stimulated Emission of Radiation.

The molecules in the lasing medium exist in an unexcited ground state. Exposure to an energy source causes stimulation of the molecules, which subsequently decay back to ground state. As a molecule decays, a photon of light energy is emitted (random emission).

The released photon is reflected in an optical resonator into the lasing medium where it collides with another excited molecule, causing the release of a photon as the molecule decays to ground state. The released photon is parallel, coherent and of the same wavelength (monochromatic) as the stimulating photon. Amplification of light energy occurs as the released photons excite further molecules, releasing more photons. The output is of high intensity light energy over a small area, despite a low initial excitation power source. This process of releasing light energy is called stimulated emission.

The lasing energy is delivered via a fibreoptic tube consisting of a series of mirrors that reflect the light and deliver it to the target. When light strikes tissues it is deflected, scattered, transmitted to deep tissues or absorbed. When the absorbed light is converted to heat, the clinical effect is seen.

Further reading

Kitching A, Edge CJ. Lasers and surgery. *Contin Educ Anaesth Crit Care Pain*. 2003; (8)5: 143–146.

24A: False
24B: False
24C: False
24D: False
24E: False
Magnetic resonance imaging uses the interaction between hydrogen molecules in the body tissues and a superimposed magnetic field to produce images of the body. MRI produces a good image of soft tissue, in multiple views, displaying blood flow and does not use ionizing radiation.

Principles of MRI

Charged particles in the nuclei of atoms in the body spin at a natural frequency, giving the atoms magnetic properties. The application of a high-powered magnetic field causes the nuclei of all these atoms to spin in alignment with this field. The MRI then applies pulses of electromagnetic radiofrequency perpendicular to the main magnetic field, which knocks the nuclei out of alignment (precession of the nuclei), producing a new magnetic field. This precession then decays and the individual nuclei emit electromagnetic waves (at individual frequencies, the Larmor frequency for that nucleus), which are detected by the MRI scanner to produce an image. The radiofrequency pulse is set to a characteristic value to hydrogen, as this is the most abundant ion in the body tissues.

Superconducting magnet

The magnetic field is generated by a superconducting electromagnet that produces a field more than 10 000 times stronger than the earth's magnetic field. When a magnetic field power is increased above 0.5 Tesla, power is dissipated in the windings of the magnet, resistance builds in the conducting elements and heat is produced. Superconductivity is the process of cooling metals to reduce electrical resistance. The superconducting magnet is cooled to near absolute zero by immersion in liquid helium (which has a boiling point of below 4.3 kelvin). As liquid helium is expensive, in practice liquid nitrogen is added to reduce the temperature of gaseous helium to below its boiling point. The magnet can be easily ramped down in emergency situations, rather than switched off. In a life-threatening emergency, the magnet can also be 'quenched', in which the coolant is vented off and the magnet may be damaged. The vent reaches extremely low temperatures and in the event of vent failure the coolant will expand, causing hypothermia and asphyxiation to anyone in the room. Note that a residual magnetic field may still be present after a quench. The cost of reactivating a magnet after a quench is considerable.

Further reading

Davis P, Kenny C. *Basic Physics and Measurement in Anaesthesia.* 5th ed. Oxford: Butterworth-Heinemann; 2003.

Reddy U, White MJ, Wilson SR. Anaesthesia for magnetic resonance imaging. *Contin Educ Anaesth Crit Care Pain.* 2012; 12(3): 140–144.

Smith T, Pinnock C, Lin T. *Fundamentals of Anaesthesia.* 3rd ed. Cambridge: Cambridge University Press; 2009.

25A: True
25B: False
25C: False
25D: True
25E: True

Permanent cardiac pacemakers are common, and present a number of safety considerations for the anaesthetist. Firstly, the underlying reason for their insertion: indications include acquired atrioventricular block, ventricular pauses and sustained ventricular tachycardia shown to be responsive to overdrive pacing.

Pacemakers tend to be located below the left clavicle and consist of a battery-powered box containing a microprocessor, with one or two leads leading to the myocardium able to sense and deliver electrical activity. If the energy applied between the anode and cathode exceeds myocardial threshold potential, cells will depolarize.

Modern pacemakers contain an anode and cathode in close proximity as opposed to older, monopolar pacemakers, where the box acted as the anode. Bipolar pacemakers are less susceptible to interference.

The functioning of cardiac pacemakers can be altered by electromagnetic interference, most commonly radiofrequency or microwaves. Magnetic resonance imaging is contraindicated. Sources of interference include:

- Monopolar diathermy: should be avoided or used well away from the pacemaker
- Mobile phones: should not be placed directly over the pacemaker but are otherwise safe
- Lithotripsy: should be at least 6 inches from pacemaker and timed with ECG
- Peripheral nerve stimulators and TENS: place away from pacemaker and not in vector with pacemaker current
- Patient shivering and positive pressure ventilation: can cause lead displacement
- Defibrillation: can cause resetting and damage but low risk if away from pacemaker site

Further reading

Diprose P, Pierce JMT. Anaesthesia for patients with pacemakers and similar devices. *Contin Educ Anaesth Crit Care Pain*. 2001; 1(6): 166–170.

26A: True
26B: True
26C: False
26D: False
26E: False

Anaesthetic scavenging systems are required to transport waste anaesthetic gases, including volatile anaesthetic agents, from the breathing system to a remote location to prevent contamination of the theatre environment.

Scavenging systems are composed of:

- Collecting system: collects waste gases from the breathing circuit
- Transfer system: hosing connecting collecting system to receiving system
- Receiving system: reservoir to store surges in waste gas flow
- Disposal system: transports waste to safe outside location (e.g. roof)

Scavenging systems can be classified as passive, whereby waste gas flow through the disposal system is powered by patient's exhalation only, or active, where sub-atmospheric pressure is generated to transmit waste gas through the disposal system.

In order to remove waste gas from expiratory flow with flow rates of 30–120 L·min^{-1}, active scavenging must be used. This employs a high-volume, low-pressure vacuum system, in contrast to the low-volume, high-pressure system used in suctioning. Therefore, the medical vacuum system used for suction is not appropriate.

Further reading

Davey AJ, Diba A. *Ward's Anaesthetic Equipment*. 5th ed. Philadelphia: Elsevier Saunders; 2005. Chapter 20, p. 401–406.

27A: False
27B: False
27C: False
27D: True
27E: False

Pulse oximetry works by spectrophotometric measurement of haemoglobin oxygen saturation. Passing radiation through a sample allows the measurement of a compound of interest by determining the quantity of radiation absorbed by that compound. Two laws describe how radiation is absorbed as it passes through a sample:

- Beer's law: the absorbance of light passing through a medium is proportional to the concentration of the medium
- Lambert's law: the absorbance of light passing through a medium is proportional to the path length (or thickness of substance)

In the pulse oximeter, light absorbed by blood depends on the quantities of deoxygenated and oxygenated haemoglobin present and the wavelength of light. At 660 nanometres wavelength (red spectrum), deoxygenated haemoglobin absorbs more light than oxygenated haemoglobin (hence red appearance of well oxygenated blood). At 940 nanometres (infrared spectrum), absorption by oxyhaemoglobin is greater than by deoxyhaemoglobin. Comparison of absorbances at these wavelengths allows pulse oximetry to calculate percentage haemoglobin oxygen saturation. The isobestic point is the point at which absorbance for oxy- and deoxyhaemoglobin is identical (805 nanometres in the infrared spectrum).

The pulse oximeter is accurate to ±2% between 70 and 100% haemoglobin oxygen saturation. Hypoperfusion, reduced cardiac output, arrhythmias and movement cause inaccurate measurements. Methaemoglobin causes a falsely low reading as it absorbs light in a similar spectrum to deoxygenated haemoglobin.

Further reading

Davis PD. *Basic Physics and Measurement in Anaesthesia*. 5th ed. Oxford: Butterworth-Heinemann; 2003.

28A: False
28B: False
28C: True
28D: False
28E: True

The centralized vacuum system consists of a pump, receiver and filter. The pump generates a negative pressure of up to –53 kPa and accommodates airflow rates of up to 40 L·min^{-1}. It is recommended that there are two outlets per operating theatre, one per anaesthetic room and one per recovery bed. A safety feature of the piped medical gas and vacuum supply outlets is by three methods of identification – colour coding, shape of outlet and the name of the gas/vacuum. The colour coding system is standardized in the UK:

- White: oxygen
- Blue: nitrous oxide
- Black: air
- Yellow: suction
- Yellow and blue: scavenging

Alternative suction systems are the mechanical foot pump or hand-held device, which is used in resuscitation and field anaesthesia, or the Venturi device, which uses a driving gas such as oxygen at flow rates of 20 L·min^{-1} (therefore it is expensive) to create a suction system.

Further reading

Al-Shaikh B, Stacey, S. *Essentials of Anaesthetic Equipment*. 2nd ed. Edinburgh: Churchill Livingstone; 2002.

29A: True
29B: True
29C: False
29D: False
29E: True
Using distilled water, at a temperature of 22°C and under a pressure of 10 kPa, the flow through 110 cm tubing with an internal diameter of 4 mm is:

- 20G: 40–80 ml·min^{-1}
- 18G: 75–120 ml·min^{-1}
- 16G: 130–220 ml·min^{-1}
- 14G: 250–360 ml·min^{-1}

Further reading

McPherson D, Adekanye O, Wilkes A, Hall JE. Fluid flow through intravenous cannulae in a clinical model. *Anesth Analg.* 2009 Apr; 108(4): 1198–1202.

30A: False
30B: False
30C: True
30D: False
30E: True
An inductor is composed of a core of ferrous material around which a conductor is tightly coiled. When a current flows along the conductor, a highly concentrated magnetic field is produced along the axis of the inductor. Applying a voltage across an inductor does not cause current to flow immediately but instead it builds up in step with the magnetic lines of force. Similarly, if the voltage is switched off, the current will slowly die away. The result is the delay in changes in current flow when a voltage varies and the prevention of surges in current.

The unit of inductance is the henry (symbol H, or L). Inductors have low resistance to DC signals and high reactance to AC signals. The impedance of an inductor is directly proportional to the frequency of AC current. Inductors are used in the defibrillator circuit to prolong the delivery of the pulse of energy to the myocardium.

Further reading

Smith T, Pinnock C, Lin T. *Fundamentals of Anaesthesia.* 3rd ed. Cambridge: Cambridge University Press; 2009. p. 253–258.

31A: False
31B: False
31C: True
31D: True
31E: False
The four laws of thermodynamics define fundamental physical quantities (temperature, energy and entropy) that characterize thermodynamic systems. The laws describe how these quantities behave under various circumstances.

The four laws of thermodynamics (and simplifications by C.P. Snow) are:

- Zeroth law of thermodynamics: if two systems are in thermal equilibrium with a third system, they must be in thermal equilibrium with each other (the triple point). This law helps define the notion of temperature, where 1 kelvin is 1/273.16 of the thermodynamic triple point of water. 'You must play the game'.
- First law of thermodynamics: heat and work are forms of energy transfer. While energy is invariably conserved, the internal energy of a closed system changes as heat and work are transferred in or out of it. Energy can neither be created nor destroyed; it can only be converted from one form to another. 'You can't win': you cannot get something for nothing, because matter and energy are conserved.
- Second law of thermodynamics: isolated systems spontaneously evolve towards thermal equilibrium. Energy will disperse from a concentrated form to a dilute form if not hindered from doing so (e.g. an anaesthetized patient will cool down in an operating theatre). 'You can't break even': you cannot return to the same energy state, because there is always an increase in disorder; entropy always increases.
- Third law of thermodynamics: the entropy of a system approaches a constant value as the temperature approaches zero. The entropy of a system at absolute zero is typically zero. 'You can't quit the game': because absolute zero is unattainable.

There are four laws but no fourth law. Although the concept of thermodynamic equilibrium is fundamental to thermodynamics, the need to state it explicitly as a law was not widely perceived until Fowler and Planck stated it in the 1930s, long after the first, second and third law were already widely understood and recognized. Hence it was numbered the zeroth law.

Further reading

Sullivan G, Edmondson C. Heat and temperature. *Contin Educ Anaesth Crit Care Pain*. 2008; 8: 104–107.

32A: True
32B: True
32C: False
32D: False
32E: True
Paramagnetic oxygen analyzers are used most frequently in theatres to measure oxygen concentration. This type of analyzer uses the principle that oxygen, together with nitric oxide, is strongly paramagnetic. This property is due to unpaired electrons in the outer shell of the atom, which is related to the atomic number of oxygen in its unionized form. In comparison, the other gases usually found in the operating theatre are weakly paramagnetic.

Infrared absorption spectroscopy relies on the fact that molecules with differing atoms (diatomic) will absorb infrared radiation at a particular wavelength. This principle can be used to measure the concentration of these diatomic molecules (e.g. carbon dioxide) in a mixture of gas. Oxygen cannot be measured with this technique.

Blood gas analysis is usually performed using a Clarke electrode for measuring oxygen, a Severinghaus electrode for carbon dioxide and a glass electrode for pH. Mass spectrometers ionize a gas sample and then accelerate the molecules using magnets, where they are separated according to their differing mass and charge. They strike a photo-voltaic detector. The mass spectrometer is very accurate and requires only small amounts of sample but is bulky and does not return the sample to the patient. The mass spectrometer is not cost effective for theatre use and is more commonly seen in a research laboratory.

Further reading

Langton JA, Hutton A. Respiratory gas analysis. *Contin Educ Anaesth Crit Care Pain.* 2009; 9: 19–23.

33A: False
33B: True
33C: True
33D: False
33E: True

NIST stands for non-interchangeable screw thread. The gas hose has a unique profile for a specific gas, which unites with the socket specific for that gas on the machine. Cylinders use the pin index system to ensure gas specific connection. The Schrader valve allows gas-specific connection with the wall pipeline system. The pressure in the pipeline is regulated to 4 bar. There are specific colours used to denote the gas that a cylinder contains or a hose carries. Oxygen is white, nitrous oxide is French blue and air is black/white.

Further reading

Sinclair C, Thadsad M, Barker I. Modern anaesthetic machines. *Contin Educ Anaesth Crit Care Pain.* 2006; 6: 75–78.

34A: False
34B: True
34C: False
34D: True
34E: True

Invasive blood pressure monitoring is the gold standard of blood pressure measurement. It not only gives you beat-to-beat information, it also allows blood sampling for blood gases and laboratory analysis. The benefit over non-invasive measurement is that it is not affected by obesity, arrhythmias or non-pulsatile flow, such as in cardiopulmonary bypass. The components in a system are an intra-arterial cannula, tubing, infusion system, transducer, microprocessor and display, mechanism for zeroing and calibration. The cannula should be short and non-tapering. The infusion system uses either a saline or heparinized saline infusion at a rate of 2–4 ml·h^{-1}. This reduces thrombus formation. The transducer should be kept level with the patient at the level of the right atrium. If the transducer is raised or lowered relative to the patient, the reading will be inaccurate. Atmospheric pressure is equal to approximately 1020 cmH$_2$O or 760 mmHg, therefore 10 cmH$_2$O is equivalent to approximately 7.5 mmHg. A 10 cm change in height will alter the pressure reading by 7.5 mmHg.

Further reading

Ward M, Langton J. Blood pressure measurement. *Contin Educ Anaesth Crit Care Pain.* 2007; 7: 122–126.

35A: False
35B: False
35C: True
35D: False
35E: True
The contents of gas cylinders are identified by clearly marked labels and a colour code. The standard used is ISO 32:1977 and states that the colour for oxygen is black with a white top, nitrous oxide is French blue and carbon dioxide is grey.

The disc around the neck of the cylinder gives the year when the cylinder was last examined and is denoted by its shape and colour.

NIST stands for non-interchangeable screw thread and is a system to prevent the wrong gas piping being attached to the wrong gas port on the anaesthetic machine. The cylinder uses a pin index system to prevent the same thing from happening.

Entonox™ cylinders if allowed to cool to below 5.5°C may begin to separate into a top layer of oxygen and a bottom layer of nitrous oxide. This may lead to a hypoxic gas mixture being vented once the top layer of oxygen has been used. Oxygen cylinders have a gauge pressure of 137 bar and an absolute pressure of 138 bar.

Further reading

Davis PD, Kenny GN. *Basic Physics and Measurement in Anaesthesia.* Oxford: Butterworth-Heinemann; 2003.

36A: False
36B: True
36C: True
36D: False
36E: False
The nerve stimulator is battery operated and should deliver a constant current up to 80 mA. It is better to deliver a constant current rather than a constant voltage as the resistance changes and this would alter the current if the stimulator supplied a constant voltage. The factor determining whether a nerve depolarizes is the current magnitude. Skin resistance is affected by skin temperature, sweat, electrode placement and in some medical conditions. Diabetes mellitus and chronic renal failure will affect the resistance too.

Other ways to measure neuromuscular blockade more accurately include: mechanomyography (MMG), electromyography (EMG) and acceleromyography. MMG measure evokes muscle tension. A muscle, usually the adductor pollicis, is held fixed under tension. The muscle is stimulated and the change in muscle tension is measured. This is felt to be the gold standard. EMG uses stimulating electrodes and recording electrodes to measure muscle action potential after stimulation of the supplying nerve. Three recording electrodes are used. EMG is prone to interference particularly from diathermy use. Acceleromyography is the technique used by the TOF Watch machine and measures the acceleration of the thumb during stimulation. Newton's second law (Force = Mass × Acceleration) is used to calculate the force of contraction.

Further reading

McGrath CD, Hunter JM. Monitoring of neuromuscular block. *Contin Educ Anaesth Crit Care Pain.* 2006; 6(1): 7–12.

37A: True
37B: True
37C: True
37D: True
37E: True
The normal distribution is also known as the Gaussian distribution or informally as the 'bell curve'. It is an example of a parametric distribution, meaning that the curve can be defined by the two parameters: the mean and the standard deviation (SD).

When the mean equals 0 and the SD is 1 the distribution is termed the standard normal deviation. The mean, mode and median all share the same value.

In a normal distribution, 2/3 of the data will lie within ±1 SD of the mean, 95% of the data lies within ±2 SD of the mean and 99.7% within ±3 SD of the mean. Skewness refers to the shape of the frequency curve. If the curve is positively skewed there will be a longer upper tail and the mean and median will be higher in value than the mode. The reverse is true if the curve is negatively skewed.

Further reading

McCluskey A, Lalkhen AG. Statistics II: central tendency and spread of data. *Contin Educ Anaesth Crit Care Pain.* 2007; 7(4): 127–130.

38A: True
38B: True
38C: False
38D: True
38E: True
There are different types of data used in statistics. The main distinction is quantitative or qualitative data, for example, height versus hair colour.

Quantitative data is continuous and is known as interval data. A subtype is integer data where the data is continuous but can only be assigned an integer value, for example, number of polyps or lymph nodes.

Non-interval data is categorical, qualitative and discrete and has two subtypes: nominal and ordinal.

Nominal means 'name' so refers to data such as hair colour or Christian names.

Ordinal data is categorical but a rank order can be applied to the categories. Arithmetic rules do not apply to the data though (e.g. pain scores, it is meaningless to say that a pain score of 4 is twice that of two and four times that of one). Ordinal data is thus pseudo-quantitative.

Further reading

McCluskey A, Lalkhen AG. Statistics I: data and correlations. *Contin Educ Anaesth Crit Care Pain.* 2007; 7(3): 95–99.

39A: False
39B: False
39C: True
39D: False
39E: False

There are various properties of solutions that depend on the osmolarity of the solution. These are referred to as the colligative properties of the solution. They depend upon the ratio of the number of solute particles to the number of solvent particles in a solution. The properties are independent of the nature of the solute particles but are due to the number of them.

Osmolarity is a term used to describe the sum total of molarities of all the solutes in a solution that give rise to the osmotic pressure.

The presence of dissolved substances, or solutes, in a solvent has a number of effects.

- Increasing the osmotic pressure
- Depression of freezing point
- Reduction of vapour pressure
- Elevation of boiling point

Raoult's law states that the reduction in vapour pressure of a solvent is proportional to the molar concentration of the solute. Consequently, the boiling point of that solvent is also elevated.

Further reading

Davis PD, Kenny GNC. *Basic Physics and Measurement in Anaesthesia.* 5th ed. Oxford: Butterworth-Heinemann; 2003. Chapter 7, p. 84–85.

40A: True
40B: True
40C: False
40D: False
40E: True

Attractive forces exist in all directions between molecules in a liquid. In the surface layer of molecules in a liquid, some of these attractive forces act in a direction parallel to the surface of the liquid. This is known as surface tension.

Surface tension can be measured as the sum of the forces acting between the molecules on either side of an imaginary straight line on the surface of the liquid. It can be expressed as force per unit length.

Surface tension is present at any air–liquid interface. In a spherical shape, such as an alveolus in the lung, the pressure created within the sphere is related to the surface tension by LaPlace's law:

$$\text{Pressure gradient across wall of a sphere} = (2 \times \text{Tension})/\text{Radius}$$

So, in smaller alveoli, the tendency will be for the pressure gradient to be so great as to cause alveolar collapse. This is reduced by the presence of surfactant. In reality, as there are two air–liquid interfaces present within an alveolus, the resulting pressure gradient is actually additive.

Further reading

Davis PD, Kenny GNC. *Basic Physics and Measurement in Anaesthesia.* 5th ed. Oxford: Butterworth-Heinemann; 2003. p. 5–18.

41A: True
41B: True
41C: False
41D: True
41E: True
Calcium is the third most abundant physiological cation and is normally found in plasma concentrations of 2.20–2.60 mmol·L^{-1}. It exists in the plasma as free ions, bound to plasma proteins such as albumin and as diffusible complexes. Calcium homeostasis is maintained by regulating absorption of calcium from the gastrointestinal tract with renal excretion as well as storage in bones, from which it can also be mobilized when required. Calcium homeostasis is regulated by three hormone systems.

Parathyroid hormone, a polypeptide secreted by the chief cells of the parathyroid gland, is affected directly by low circulating calcium and acts to increase plasma calcium levels. Calcitonin, in contrast, acts to lower plasma calcium levels and is secreted by the parafollicular cells of the thyroid gland. The vitamin D group of sterols also plays a vital role in regulating plasma calcium levels.

Further reading

Khan MM, Desborough JP. Calcium homeostasis. *Update in Anaesthesia.* 2005; 19(7): 1.

Parikh M, Webb ST. Cations: potassium, calcium and magnesium. *Contin Educ Anaesth Crit Care Pain.* 2012; 12(4): 195–198.

42A: True
42B: True
42C: False
42D: True
42E: False

Bicarbonate (HCO_3^-) forms the main physiological buffer system, serving to maintain plasma pH within the normal range of 7.35–7.45. Plasma bicarbonate is freely filtered at the glomerulus, and 99% is reabsorbed by the kidney at normal plasma concentrations. The majority (90%) is reabsorbed in the proximal convoluted tubule as carbon dioxide and water following the formation of carbonic acid (H_2CO_3) by combination with H^+ ions secreted into the urine.

$$HCO_3^- + H^+ \rightleftharpoons H_2CO_3 \rightleftharpoons CO_2 + H_2O$$

If plasma levels of bicarbonate exceed the tubular (or 'transport') maximum (Tm; the highest rate at which renal tubules may transport a substance, after which it may be excreted in urine), then bicarbonate is lost in the urine, which becomes more alkaline. In the distal convoluted tubule and collecting duct, the remainder of bicarbonate is reabsorbed, again as carbon dioxide and water from carbonic acid, following H^+ secretion by the H^+/K^+ ATPase and Na^+/H^+ exchange transporters.

Further reading

Kitching AJ, Edge CJ. Acid-base balance: a review of normal physiology. *Contin Educ Anaesth Crit Care Pain*. 2002; 2(1): 3–6.

Rassam SS, Counsel DJ. Perioperative electrolyte and fluid balance. *Contin Educ Anaesth Crit Care Pain*. 2005; 5(5): 157–160.

43A: True
43B: False
43C: False
43D: True
43E: False
Functional residual capacity (FRC) is the sum of the residual volume (RV) and the expiratory reserve volume (ERV). It is the volume remaining in the lungs at the end of expiration during normal tidal breathing. Normal FRC lies on the steepest part of the lung compliance curve, and is also associated with minimal pulmonary vascular resistance. The FRC is normally approximately 2500 ml in an adult male (1800 in an adult female) but is reduced in conditions that displace the diaphragm cephalad, such as pregnancy or abdominal distension, as well as those which reduce RV, such as fibrotic lung disease or restrictive chest wall defects. In addition, lying supine will reduce the FRC as does general anaesthesia. As the FRC includes the RV, it cannot be measured by simple spirometry, but can be derived by body plethysmography or helium dilution.

Further reading

West JB. *Respiratory Physiology: The Essentials*. 8th ed. Philadelphia: Lippincott Williams & Wilkins; 2008.

Wild M, Alagesan K. PEEP and CPAP. *Contin Educ Anaesth Crit Care Pain*. 2001; 1(3): 89–92.

44A: False
44B: True
44C: False
44D: True
44E: True

Hypoxic pulmonary vasoconstriction (HPV) is an active process affecting pulmonary blood flow. It occurs in response to reduced partial pressure of alveolar oxygen (P_AO_2), causing constriction of small pulmonary arteries and diverting blood flow away from poorly ventilated portions of lung. This reduces the shunt fraction of cardiac output by preferentially perfusing better ventilated areas. The exact mechanism of HPV is not clear but it has been demonstrated to occur in excised portions of lung tissue and therefore is not thought to be dependent on central nervous system control. A number of factors can alter the HPV response: it is inhibited by drugs that cause vasodilation such as glyceryl trinitrate, as well as by volatile anaesthetic agents, but not the intravenous anaesthetic agents such as propofol and thiopental.

Further reading

Eastwood J, Mahajan R. One-lung anaesthesia. *Contin Educ Anaesth Crit Care Pain*. 2002; 2(3): 83–87.

Hills GH. Respiratory physiology and anaesthesia. *Contin Educ Anaesth Crit Care Pain*. 2001; 1(2): 35–39.

45A: True
45B: True
45C: False
45D: True
45E: True

Polycythaemia refers to haemoglobin concentrations above the normal range for that individual. It can occur due to primary or secondary causes.

Primary polycythaemia (e.g. polycythaemia vera) results from a genetic anomaly in erythroblastic cells leading to excessive erythrocyte production.

Secondary polycythaemia is caused by increased erythropoiesis in response to low arterial oxygen levels, such as those seen in impaired oxygen delivery (e.g. chronic heart or lung disease) or low fractions of inspired oxygen (e.g. high altitude). Polycythaemia seen in people living at high altitude is known as physiological polycythaemia.

Physiological effects of polycythaemia include:

- Increase in haematocrit
- Increase in total blood volume (seen in polycythaemia vera)
  - Vascular engorgement
  - Increases venous return
- Increase in blood viscosity
  - Reduction in peripheral blood flow
  - Cyanosis due to increased concentration of deoxygenated haemoglobin
  - Decreased cardiac venous return

- Relatively normal cardiac output
  - Due to opposing factors on venous return
- Hypertension
  - In one-third of patients due to vasoconstriction and increased total blood volume

Further reading

Guyton AC, Hall JE. *Textbook of Medical Physiology*. 11th ed. Philadelphia: Elsevier Saunders; 2006.

Miller RD (Ed). *Miller's Anaesthesia*. 6th ed. Philadelphia: Elsevier; 2005.

46A: False
46B: True
46C: False
46D: True
46E: True

Intermittent positive pressure ventilation (IPPV) is indicated in anaesthesia for many types of surgery, and the decision regarding its use relies on many factors, including the need for muscle relaxation, location of surgery, likely access to the airway and duration and extent of the operation.

The change from spontaneous ventilation, involving generation of negative intrathoracic pressure to draw air into the lungs, to positive pressure ventilation, forcing air into the lungs, causes some changes in physiology.

Cardiovascular changes are mostly related to changes in intrathoracic pressure. Increases in intrathoracic pressure during inspiration can lead to a decrease in cardiac output. It increases right atrial pressure and therefore reduces the pressure gradient for venous return. This reduces right ventricular filling. The increased intrathoracic pressure also decreases left ventricular afterload by decreasing left ventricular transmural pressure but this beneficial effect is counteracted by the reduction in preload, and an increase in pulmonary vascular resistance, which increases right ventricular afterload and therefore limits left ventricular filling.

Respiratory changes can be both beneficial and detrimental. Positive end expiratory pressure (PEEP) can significantly reduce the work of breathing and improves oxygenation by recruitment of alveoli in previously poorly ventilated areas of the lung but preferential ventilation of poorly perfused areas of lung will increase ventilation/perfusion (V/Q) mismatching. If cardiac output falls as described earlier, pulmonary perfusion will be reduced, increasing alveolar dead space and further contributing to V/Q mismatch. Prolonged IPPV also reduces secretion of surfactant. Increases in alveolar distension can be beneficial but can also result in barotrauma, over distension and damage to alveolar epithelium due to repeated opening and closing of collapsed alveoli (atalectrauma).

Further reading

McConachie I. *Handbook of ICU Therapy*. 2nd ed. Cambridge: Cambridge University Press; 2006. p. 113–116.

Smith T, Pinnock C, Lin T. *Fundamentals of Anaesthesia*. 3rd ed. Cambridge: Cambridge University Press; 2009.

47A: False
47B: False
47C: True
47D: True
47E: False

Many physiological changes of importance to the anaesthetist take place during the course of pregnancy. Increased oedema and capillary engorgement of the upper airway as well as breast engorgement can make direct laryngoscopy more difficult in the pregnant patient.

Cephalad displacement of the diaphragm by the gravid uterus results in a 20% reduction in functional residual capacity (FRC) at term. Combined with an increased metabolic rate and oxygen consumption, the time to desaturation following apnoea is reduced. FRC may well encroach on closing capacity in the third trimester, reducing the effectiveness of preoxygenation and compounding this effect.

Other respiratory changes include an increase in minute ventilation due to both a progesterone-mediated increase in respiratory rate, as well as an increased tidal volume. This reduces arterial $PaCO_2$ to 4.1 kPa by the third trimester.

Progesterone and oestrogen-mediated increase in renin production by the kidney results in a 45% increase in plasma volume. Despite an increase in red cell mass, dilutional anaemia of pregnancy is also seen due to the greater increase in plasma volume. These hormones also lead to vasodilatation and a resulting fall in systemic vascular resistance. Cardiac output is increased by 50% at term due to an increase in heart rate and stroke volume. This compensates somewhat for the increase in oxygen demand. No increase in contractility is seen, although left ventricular dilatation and hypertrophy may occur.

Renal plasma flow and glomerular filtration rate increase during pregnancy, and lower oesophageal sphincter incompetence is seen due to progesterone-mediated smooth muscle relaxation. Combined with reduced gastric emptying seen during labour means that the risk of aspiration during general anaesthesia is significant. Plasma concentrations of clotting factors increase, with the exception of XI and XIII, leading to a hypercoagulable state.

Further reading

Heidemann BH, McClure JH. Changes in maternal physiology during pregnancy. *Contin Educ Anaesth Crit Care Pain*. 2003; 3(3): 65–68.

48A: True
48B: True
48C: False
48D: False
48E: False

Progressive physiological changes are seen with advancing age, distinct from those associated with disease processes. They affect all body systems, and usually reflect a decline in function.

Cardiac output, heart rate and stroke volume are reduced, as is left ventricular compliance. A reduction in vital capacity is seen, along with an increase in residual volume and consequent reduction in functional residual capacity. Chest wall compliance is reduced but lung elasticity is also reduced, increasing lung compliance.

A decline in renal mass and concentrating ability is seen as well as a reduced renal response to vasopressin. Brain mass is reduced and there is a reduction in cerebral blood flow.

Several theories have been proposed for this age-related decline in physiological function but at present it remains incompletely understood.

Further reading

Murray D, Dodds C. Perioperative care of the elderly. *Contin Educ Anaesth Crit Care Pain.* 2004; 4(6): 193–196.

Schofield P. 'It's your age': the assessment and management of pain in older adults. *Contin Educ Anaesth Crit Care Pain.* 2010; 10(3): 93–95.

49A: False
49B: True
49C: False
49D: True
49E: True

The primary function of the lung is to allow blood to come into contact with atmospheric air for gas exchange to occur; though it has a number of other functions too. It acts as a reservoir of blood and filters small thrombi before they enter the circulation of other organs. As the lungs receive all of the circulating volume together with the heart, it metabolizes a number of vasoactive substances. The following table shows the fate of a number of substances in the pulmonary circulation.

Substance	Metabolism
Peptides	
Angiotensin I	Converted to angiotensin II by ACE
Angiotensin II	Unaffected
Vasopressin	Unaffected
Bradykinin	Up to 80% inactivated
Amines	
Serotonin	Almost completely removed
Noradrenaline	Up to 30% removed
Histamine	Unaffected
Dopamine	Unaffected
Arachidonic Acid Metabolites	
Prostaglandin E_2 and $F_{2\alpha}$	Almost completely removed
Prostaglandin A_2	Unaffected
Prostacyclin (PGI_2)	Unaffected
Leukotrienes	Almost completely removed

Further reading

West JB. *Respiratory Physiology: The Essentials*. 9th ed. Philadelphia: Lippincott Williams & Wilkins; 2011.

50A: False
50B: False
50C: True
50D: True
50E: False
Haem is an iron-porphyrin compound that combines to a globin protein to form haemoglobin. The protein globin is composed of four polypeptide chains. In an adult these are two α- and two β-chains. Normal haemoglobin A (HbA) can have its iron component oxidized. When the ferrous ion is oxidized to its ferric form it is called methaemoglobin (MetHb).

Oxygen combines easily with haemoglobin to form oxyhaemoglobin. The amount of haemoglobin that is converted to oxyhaemoglobin depends on the partial pressure of oxygen that haemoglobin is exposed to. This is represented graphically by the oxygen dissociation curve. The oxygen dissociation curve is shifted to the right by an increase in H^+ concentration (or decrease in pH), PCO_2, temperature and concentration of 2,3-diphosphoglycerate (2,3 DPG). Haemoglobin also has an affinity for carbon monoxide, which is around 240 times stronger than for oxygen.

Haemoglobin will also bind hydrogen ions and carbon dioxide. This occurs more avidly when the haemoglobin is in its deoxygenated rather than oxygenated state.

Further reading

Thomas C, Lumb A. Physiology of haemoglobin. *Contin Educ Anaesth Crit Care Pain*. 2012; 12(5): 251–256.

51A: False
51B: False
51C: True
51D: True
51E: True
The pathways transmitting pain sensation during labour vary according to the site of origin of the pain and the stage of labour.

The uterus, lower uterine segment and cervix are all supplied by afferent Aδ and C fibres. They accompany the sacral and thoracolumbar sympathetic outflow. The pain of the first stage of labour is transmitted through these pathways as stretching and dilatation of the uterus and cervix occurs. Pain in the first stage of labour is poorly localized and referred initially to the dermatomes of T10 to L1. As labour progresses, descent of the foetal head leads to pain referred to the lower lumbar and sacral dermatomes.

As labour enters the second stage there is additional pain arising from the stretching of perineal structures. This involves somatic pain sensation, which is better localized and transmitted again in Aδ and C fibres via the pudendal nerves and S2–4 nerve roots to the spinal cord.

Further reading

Yentis S, May A, Malhotra S. *Analgesia, Anaesthesia and Pregnancy: A Practical Guide.* 2nd ed. Cambridge: Cambridge University Press; 2007.

52A: False
52B: True
52C: False
52D: False
52E: True
The diaphragmatic surface, or base, of the heart is composed of both the right and left ventricles together with the portion of the right atrium that receives the inferior vena cava.

The right atrium is larger than the left atrium but somewhat thinner walled. The right atrium receives the superior vena cava in its upper and posterior part; the inferior vena cava and coronary sinus in its lower part. The anterior cardiac vein enters anteriorly.

The moderator band is a muscular structure crossing the right ventricle from the interventricular septum to the anterior wall. It conveys the right branch of the atrioventricular bundle.

Lying above the three semilunar cusps of the aortic valve are the dilated aortic sinuses. These are the anterior, left posterior and right posterior. The origins of the right coronary and left coronary artery are seen within the anterior and left posterior sinuses, respectively.

Further reading

Ellis H, Feldman S, Harrop-Griffiths W. *Anatomy for Anaesthetists.* 8th ed. Oxford: Wiley-Blackwell; 2003.

53A: True
53B: False
53C: False
53D: True
53E: True
Cerebrospinal fluid (CSF) is the clear fluid that fills the cerebral ventricles and the subarachnoid space. Total volume is approximately 150 ml with 25 ml of that held within the spine.

CSF is produced by the choroid plexus of the lateral, third and fourth ventricles. The CSF flows from the lateral ventricles to the third ventricle via the foramen of

Monro. It then passes from the third to the fourth ventricle via the aqueduct of Sylvius. CSF leaves the fourth ventricle via the middle foramen of Magendie and by the lateral foramina of Luschka. It is absorbed by the arachnoid granulations, which are small projections of arachnoid that pierce the dura covering the venous sinuses.

Lying in the lateral position the pressure is 70–180 mmCSF. There are no valves in the system, so, when sitting, the pressure in the lumbar region rises to 350–550 mm of CSF.

Further reading

Ellis H, Feldman S, Harrop-Griffiths W. *Anatomy for Anaesthetists*. 8th ed. Oxford: Wiley-Blackwell; 2003.

54A: True
54B: False
54C: True
54D: False
54E: True
The antecubital fossa (ACF) is a triangular area located on the volar aspect of the forearm. The boundaries are:

- Medial: pronator teres
- Laterally: brachoradialis
- Inferior: a line connecting the medial and lateral epicondyles of the humerus

The roof of the ACF is formed by deep fascia, which is reinforced by the bicipital aponeurosis. On the fascia lies the median cubital vein, a common site for venepuncture and cannulation. The median cubital vein is crossed by the medial cutaneous nerve of the forearm, occasionally damaged by venepuncture.

The contents from medial to lateral are: the median nerve, brachial artery, biceps tendon and radial nerve. The brachial artery is a site for arterial cannulation and is a large end artery. The cephalic vein drains the radial side of the forearm and lies proximally on the lateral side of the ACF and on the lateral border of the biceps muscle. The basilic vein drains the medial side of the forearm and ascends on the medial side of the biceps.

Further reading

Ellis H, Feldman S, Harrop-Griffiths W. *Anatomy for Anaesthetists*. 8th ed. Oxford: Wiley-Blackwell; 2003.

55A: True
55B: False
55C: False
55D: True
55E: True

The spinal cord is up to 45 cm in length in the adult male and originates superiorly as a continuation of the medulla oblongata at the foramen magnum and terminates at the level of L1/2 in the adult, where it tapers into the conus medullaris. The filum terminale extends inferiorly to attach to the coccyx. The spinal cord contains ascending sensory and descending motor tracts.

The dorsal columns carry fine touch, vibration and proprioception sensations. Fibres enter the cord and run in the fasciculus gracilis (medial, carries fibres from the lower body, below T6) and the cuneates fasciculus (lateral, carries fibres from the upper body, above T6). The tracts then decussate in the medulla and continue to the sensory cortex.

The spinothalamic tracts carry pain, temperature and coarse touch sensation to the thalamus and the sensory cortex. The fibres carrying this sensory information enter the cord through the dorsal route and decussate before ascending in the spinothalamic tracts.

The lateral corticospinal tract carries information from the motor cortex and decussates in the medulla before descending in the lateral aspect of the cord.

Cord hemisection (Brown-Séquard syndrome) hence will cause ipsilateral loss of fine touch, proprioception and vibration sense as well as ipsilateral motor weakness and contralateral loss of pain, temperature and coarse touch sensation.

Further reading

Power I, Kam P. *Principles of Physiology for the Anaesthetist*. 2nd ed. London: Hodder Arnold; 2008.

56A: True
56B: True
56C: True
56D: True
56E: True
The lymphatic system is formed by a network of capillaries that drain lymph into sequentially larger vessels towards the thoracic ducts. The lymphatic system drains interstitial fluid, protein and fat molecules into lymph, which is returned to the circulation. In addition, lymph absorbs proteins and molecules that have accumulated in inflamed tissue and returns them to the circulation.

Further reading

Levick JR, Michel CC. Microvascular fluid exchange and the revised Starling principle. *Cardiovascular Research*. 2010; 87(2): 198–210.

57A: True
57B: False
57C: False
57D: True
57E: False

Cerebral blood flow is 14% of the resting cardiac output and 50 ml·100 g^{-1}·min^{-1} of brain tissue. Cerebral blood flow is affected by a number of factors. Autoregulation maintains constant blood flow over a mean arterial pressure range of 50–150 mmHg by the Bayliss effect (a myogenic response to fluctuations in perfusion pressure in arterioles). Beyond these limits the relationship is linear. In the elderly and in patients with chronic hypertension, the autoregulation curve is shifted to the right. Cerebral perfusion pressure (CPP) is related to MAP and intracranial pressure (ICP) and central venous pressure (CVP) in the equation:

$$CPP = MAP - (ICP + CVP)$$

Carbon dioxide crosses the blood–brain barrier and causes arteriolar vasodilation, which leads to an increase in cerebral blood flow. This relationship is linear at normal MAP, where every 1 mmHg (0.13 kPa) rise in PaCO$_2$ causes a 2–4% rise in cerebral blood flow. At normal PaO$_2$ ranges, there is no effect on cerebral blood flow; however, hypoxia causes vasodilation when the PaO$_2$ falls below 6.7 kPa.

Further reading

Girling K. Management of head injury in the intensive-care unit. *Contin Educ Anaesth Crit Care Pain.* 2004; 4(2): 52–56.

58A: False
58B: True
58C: False
58D: False
58E: True
The concentration of hydrogen ions in the body is tightly regulated to allow enzymes, cell membranes, ATP release and reflexes to function normally. At a physiological pH of 7.4, [H$^+$] is 40 nmol·L^{-1}.

The pH scale is a negative logarithmic scale (pH = $-\log_{10}$ [H$^+$]). Hence small changes in pH reflect large changes in [H$^+$]. The Brønsted-Lowry theory defines an acid as a substance that donates a proton and a base as a substance that accepts a proton.

There are three main mechanisms of acid–base homeostasis: buffering, compensation and correction. The major buffer system in the body is the H$_2$CO$_3$ (carbonic acid)/HCO$_3^-$ (bicarbonate) buffer system. This is an open buffer system, whereby the bicarbonate, carbon dioxide and water content of the body can be adjusted by the kidneys and lungs, rendering it effective in buffering large amounts of hydrogen ions. The pKa of this system is 6.1.

Further reading

Smith T, Pinnock C, Lin T. *Fundamentals of Anaesthesia.* 3rd ed. Cambridge: Cambridge University Press; 2009. p. 253–258.

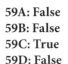

59A: False
59B: False
59C: True
59D: False
59E: True

The thyroid gland is the largest endocrine gland in the body, which, when stimulated by thyroid stimulating hormone (TSH, from the anterior pituitary), produces thyroxine (T_4) and tri-iodothyronine (T_3). Iodination of tyrosine residues on thyroglobulin forms the mono-iodotyrosine (MIT) and di-iodotyrosine (DIT), which combine to form T_3 (one molecule of MIT, one of DIT) and T_4 (two molecules of DIT). T_3 is considerably more potent and active than T_4; however, the majority (90%) of thyroid hormone production is as the T_4 form, which is converted to T_3 in the peripheral tissues. Thyroid hormones are transported in the plasma bound to thyroxine binding globulin (67%), thyroxine binding pre-albumin (20%) and albumin (13%). Thyroid hormones are steroid hormones that cross the target cell membrane to bind intracellular receptors, altering gene transcription and cellular protein production. Action of the thyroid hormones is terminated by conversion to the inactive recombinant T_3 (rT_3) in the liver.

Further reading

Malhotra S, Sodhi V. Anaesthesia for thyroid and parathyroid surgery. *Contin Educ Anaesth Crit Care Pain.* 2007; 7(2): 55–58.

60A: False
60B: True
60C: False
60D: False
60E: True

The sarcomere is the basic contractile unit of the skeletal muscle cell. It is composed of multiple protein complexes with thick and thin filaments. The thick filaments are composed of myosin molecules. Myosin has two globular heads (the ATP- and actin-binding sites), which are attached to a rod-shaped tail; the molecules are kept aligned at the M-line (for *mittelscheibe* or 'middle disc'). The thin filaments are composed of two chains of actin molecules in a helical arrangement with a tropomyosin chain lying between the grooves of the actin chains. Troponin (C, I, T-subunits) is associated with the tropomyosin. The thin filaments are kept aligned at the Z-line (*zwischenscheibe* or 'between disc').

During contraction, an action potential stimulates the myofibril causing calcium release from the sarcoplasmic reticulum. Calcium binds troponin-C, causing a conformational change in troponin-I and -T. Tropomyosin moves away from the groove, exposing actin. Myosin binds to actin, forming cross-bridges. Under the influence of ATP, the myosin head bends, causing shortening of the sarcomere (shortening of the H band; *Heller* or 'brighter').

Relaxation is an active process as calcium reuptake into the sarcoplasmic reticulum occurs by the Ca/Mg-ATPase pump. In death, *rigor mortis* occurs when the ATP is consumed and calcium reuptake cannot occur, causing persistent skeletal muscle contraction. In relaxation, troponin and tropomyosin resume their usual configuration, blocking actin once again.

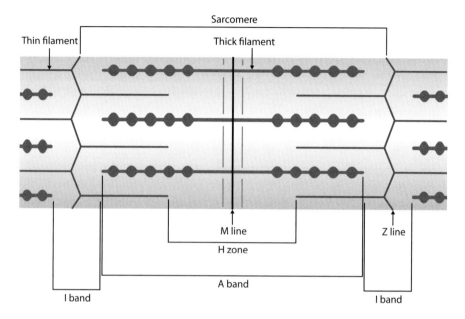

Further reading

Hopkins PM. Skeletal muscle physiology. *Contin Educ Anaesth Crit Care Pain.* 2006; 6(1): 1–6.

1. Atracurium:
  A. Undergoes Hofmann degradation by cleavage of central ester groups of the methyl chain
  B. Is broken down to the active metabolite laudanosine
  C. Undergoes ester hydrolysis primarily in the neuromuscular junction
  D. Possesses 10 chiral molecules
  E. Causes significantly prolonged neuromuscular blockade in patients with renal failure

2. Warfarin:
  A. Is highly protein-bound
  B. Inhibits the oxidation of reduced vitamin K
  C. Has low oral bioavailability
  D. Is less effective when administered with amiodarone
  E. Is eliminated largely unchanged in the urine

3. The following are correct:
  A. The $GABA_A$ receptor is a ligand-gated ion channel
  B. The $GABA_A$ receptor has a transmembrane serpentine structure
  C. Benzodiazepines bind to the alpha subunit of the $GABA_B$ receptor, increasing chloride conductance
  D. The $GABA_B$ receptor is located on the post-synaptic membrane
  E. The $GABA_B$ receptor is a G-protein-coupled receptor

4. The following statements are correct.
  A. The velocity of a substrate-enzyme reaction can be calculated using the Menton constant
  B. Insulin is a positive allosteric modulator of adenylyl cyclase
  C. A patient on rifampicin will require larger doses of warfarin to achieve a therapeutic INR
  D. The action of adrenaline at β-adrenoceptors is an example of receptor potentiation
  E. Etomidate inhibits cytochrome P450 enzymes

5. Furosemide:
A. Is an organic acid
B. Is completely cleared by the kidney
C. Has reduced efficacy in patients taking warfarin
D. Acts in the ascending limb of the loop of Henle
E. Has an elimination half-life of approximately 2 hours in healthy individuals

6. Vasopressin:
A. Is a pro-hormone
B. Has a half-life of 24 hours
C. Is a steroid hormone
D. Has a tenth of the antidiuretic action of desmopressin
E. Acts as a neurotransmitter

7. The following IV fluids have a sodium concentration that is higher than that normally found in plasma:
A. Gelofusine
B. 8.4% sodium bicarbonate
C. 20% human albumin solution
D. 0.9% sodium chloride
E. Hartmann's solution

8. Doxapram:
A. Reverses opioid-induced respiratory depression and analgesia
B. Is effective in the treatment of postoperative shivering
C. Primarily acts directly on the respiratory centre in the brainstem
D. Has a duration of action of 1–2 minutes
E. Displaces the CO_2 vs minute volume response curve to the left

9. Dexmedetomidine:
A. Causes bradycardia
B. Is an antagonist at the α_2-adrenergic receptor
C. Has MAC-sparing effects in general anaesthesia
D. Has a rapid onset of action
E. Has a variable offset of action

10. Methadone:
A. Exists as a racemic mixture
B. Is mainly bound to albumin
C. Has a short elimination period
D. Is metabolized in the liver by the P450 enzyme system
E. Is a partial μ-opioid agonist

11. Paracetamol:
A. Has significant first-pass metabolism
B. Easily crosses the blood–brain barrier and the placenta
C. Is removed by haemodialysis
D. Only inhibits the *COX-2* enzyme
E. Is absorbed faster rectally than it is orally

12. Volume of distribution:
A. Is a physiological value
B. Of propofol is 250 litres
C. Decreases with age
D. Of warfarin is 80 litres
E. Is increased in renal and liver failure

13. Bupivacaine:
A. Is 80% protein-bound
B. Has a volume of distribution of 20 to 100 L
C. Is only available as a racemic mixture
D. Is less cardio toxic when presented as the R-isomer
E. Has a pKa of 8.1

14. Sulphonylureas:
A. Are used in the treatment of type I and II diabetes mellitus
B. Increase peripheral insulin resistance
C. Reduce glucagon secretion
D. Cause pancreatic β-cell hyperplasia
E. Increase insulin production

15. The following are prodrugs:
A. Diamorphine
B. Terlipressin
C. Omeprazole
D. Captopril
E. Carbimazole

16. Drugs suitable for transdermal delivery include:
A. Buprenorphine
B. Hyoscine
C. Morphine
D. Clonidine
E. Glyceryl trinitrate

17. Carbimazole:
A. Inhibits activity of thyroid peroxidase
B. Is a prodrug
C. Has poor oral bioavailability
D. Is used to treat hypothyroidism
E. Can cross the placenta

18. Etomidate:
A. Has two chiral centres
B. May inhibit plasma cholinesterase
C. Enhances the effect of GABA at the $GABA_B$ receptor
D. Decreases intracranial pressure
E. Inhibits the baroreceptor reflex

19. **Factors increasing placental drug transfer include:**
    A. High lipid solubility
    B. Foetal acidaemia for basic drugs
    C. Foetal alkalosis for basic drugs
    D. High placental blood flow
    E. High degree of ionization

20. **The following opiates have no action at κ-opioid receptors:**
    A. Morphine
    B. Tramadol
    C. Remifentanil
    D. Pethidine
    E. Diamorphine

21. **The following sites do not correlate well with cerebral temperature:**
    A. Nasopharynx
    B. Proximal oesophagus
    C. Bladder
    D. Pulmonary artery
    E. Tympanic membrane

22. **The gas laws state that:**
    A. The inverse relationship between volume and temperature is Charles' law
    B. An ideal gas is subject to intermolecular forces
    C. At a constant volume, the absolute pressure of a given mass of gas is inversely proportional to the absolute temperature
    D. At a constant pressure, the volume of a given mass of gas is directly proportional to the absolute temperature
    E. The amount of gas dissolved in a liquid is proportional to the partial pressure of the gas above the liquid

23. **The accuracy of the thermodilution technique for measuring cardiac output can be influenced by:**
    A. Tricuspid regurgitation, causing overestimation of cardiac output
    B. Cardiac bypass
    C. Anaemia
    D. Positive pressure ventilation
    E. Pulmonary stenosis

24. **With use of ultrasound:**
    A. The frequency of sound audible to humans is 20 Hz to 20 kHz
    B. Each reflected sound wave is represented by a dot in the image on the monitor
    C. Piezoelectric crystals act as transducers by converting electrical energy into sound and vice versa
    D. Bone appears brighter than blood on the ultrasound image
    E. Medical ultrasound typically uses frequencies in the order of kilohertz

25. **The following are correct with respect to optical fibres:**
    A. Fibreoptics work on the principle of total internal reflection
    B. If the angle of incidence is less than the critical angle, light will be refracted
    C. The outer layer of a fibreoptic glass fibre has a higher refractive index
    D. The bundle of fibres in a fibreoptic laryngoscope is not coherent
    E. Light travelling in a fibreoptic laryngoscope does not pass between fibres

26. **In the use of peripheral nerve stimulators:**
    A. A single twitch comprises a supramaximal stimulus >60 mA for 0.2 s
    B. Double burst stimuli consist of two bursts of two stimuli, 750 ms apart
    C. A complete train of four takes 1500 ms
    D. Tetanic stimulation is applied at a frequency of 5 Hz
    E. Post-tetanic count should be performed 3 s after the period of tetany

27. **The following statements are correct regarding infrared spectrophotometry:**
    A. Absorbance of infrared by carbon dioxide peaks at a wavelength of 4.28 micrometres
    B. The partial pressure of nitrous oxide may be overestimated in the presence of oxygen
    C. The process works on the principle that molecules containing two or more similar atoms will absorb infrared radiation at specific wavelengths
    D. The partial pressure of carbon dioxide may be overestimated if measured in the presence of nitrous oxide
    E. Accuracy is improved by the use of a double-beamed instrument

28. **The critical temperature:**
    A. Is the temperature above which a gas can be liquefied if sufficient pressure is applied
    B. Is the temperature at which a gas mixture will separate into its constituents
    C. For nitrous oxide is 36.5°C
    D. Is the temperature at which a gas cannot be liquefied, no matter how much pressure is applied
    E. Is the temperature at which one mole of a gas occupies 22.4 litres and contains 6.02×10^{23} molecules

29. **Latent heat of vaporization:**
    A. Falls as the temperature rises
    B. Is zero when the saturated vapour pressure of water equals atmospheric pressure
    C. Is zero when a substance is at its critical temperature
    D. Is lost during humidification
    E. Is best demonstrated using an isobologram

30. **A line isolation monitor:**
    A. Is connected to earth
    B. Alarms in cases of excessive current surge through the circuit
    C. Switches off the power supply if an earth connection is made
    D. Alarms if an earth connection is made
    E. Disconnects the circuit if an earth connection is made

31. Regarding heat loss during anaesthesia:
A. A 1 litre bag of fluid at room temperature will not reduce body temperature by more than 0.1°C
B. The greatest source of heat loss is by evaporation
C. General anaesthesia can reduce body temperature by 0.5–1°C within the first hour
D. Loss of heat is by four main mechanisms: convection, evaporation, conduction and radiation
E. Heat loss during evaporation is due to the latent heat of vaporization

32. Which of the following statements about SI units are correct?
A. SI stands for Scientifique Information
B. There are two types of SI units: fundamental and derived
C. There are seven fundamental units
D. The gram is the SI unit of mass
E. The SI unit of temperature is the kelvin

33. Which of the following statements is correct regarding the desflurane TEC 6 vaporizer?
A. It is a draw-over type vaporizer
B. It contains an internal heating element
C. It contains a variable pressure transducer
D. It utilizes a bimetallic strip for temperature compensation
E. It needs a separate power source

34. Damping in an electromanometer:
A. Is optimal when the damping factor is two thirds of critical damping
B. May be increased by the presence of a clot in the line
C. Is increased as the catheter gets shorter and wider
D. Is said to be absent when the damping ratio is equal to 1
E. Helps prevents overshoot of the measured pressure in response to a step change in pressure

35. The following pairings are correct:
A. Adjustable pressure limiting valve: 5–6 kPa
B. Back bar pressure relief valve: 340 cmH_2O
C. Pipeline supply: 3000 mmHg
D. N_2O cylinder pressure: 5.5 MPa
E. O_2 cylinder pressure: 13 700 cmH_2O

36. Regarding retrospective studies:
A. They are less useful than prospective studies when investigating rare diseases
B. They are prone to recall bias
C. Cohort studies are an example of a retrospective study
D. Usually require large funds and multi-centre involvement
E. They involve randomization to an interventional or control group

37. **The null hypothesis:**
    A. Is incorrectly accepted in a type I (α) error
    B. States that there is no difference between groups for the variable of interest
    C. Is standardly rejected if the P value is less than 0.5
    D. Is incorrectly rejected in a type II (β) error
    E. Likelihood of being correctly rejected is found by $1 - \beta$

38. **When monitoring the ECG in theatre:**
    A. Lead I is best for detecting myocardial ischaemia
    B. The CM5 lead is best for detecting arrhythmias
    C. Lead II detects the potential difference between the right arm and left arm
    D. Lead III detects the potential difference between the left arm and left leg
    E. The 'M' in the CM5 lead position refers to mid-clavicular line

39. **When using pulmonary function monitoring:**
    A. Wright's peak flowmeter is a constant pressure, variable orifice device
    B. The Benedict-Roth spirometer can be used to measure total lung capacity
    C. The vitalograph plots expired volume–time graphs
    D. The Wright's respirometer can be used to measure continuous gas flow
    E. The pneumotacograph is affected by gas temperature

40. **Radiation:**
    A. Dosage is quantified in Bequerels
    B. Exposure is higher from a chest X-ray than a skull X-ray
    C. Exposure from a CT chest and abdomen confers a lifetime cancer risk of 1 in 2000
    D. Exposure from fluoroscopy is very minimal
    E. Exposure from a CT chest abdomen is equivalent to 4 years background exposure

41. **Magnesium:**
    A. Is physiologically active in its ionized form
    B. Is reabsorbed in the ascending limb of the loop of Henle
    C. Is an essential cofactor in ATP-dependent processes
    D. Is a competitive antagonist at voltage-gated calcium channels
    E. Inhibits acetylcholine release at the neuromuscular junction

42. **At the sino-atrial node:**
    A. Phase 2 of the action potential is caused by opening of L-type calcium channels
    B. Threshold potential is –50 mV
    C. Depolarization occurs due to opening of voltage-gated sodium channels
    D. Pacemaker potential is due to decreased membrane potassium permeability
    E. Vagal stimulation increases potassium permeability

43. **Physiological dead space:**
    A. Is measured using Fowler's method
    B. Is increased with supine posture
    C. Is about 150 ml in an adult male
    D. Is the volume of the conducting airways
    E. Is reduced with increasing age

44. The spirometry trace pictured depicts the following measurements:

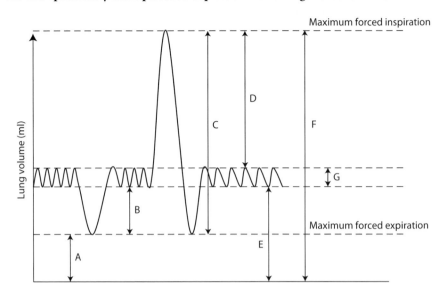

A. A is functional residual capacity
B. C is total lung capacity
C. G is tidal volume
D. E is reduced in pregnancy
E. F can be measured by simple spirometry

45. Within the neuromuscular junction:
A. A muscle cell may be innervated by multiple neuromuscular junctions
B. Binding of one acetylcholine molecule to the α-subunit opens the acetylcholine receptor
C. Acetylcholine synthesis only takes place in the cell body
D. 12 000 molecules of acetylcholine are released after each nerve impulse
E. The acetylcholine receptor is a G-protein-coupled receptor

46. Anaphylaxis:
A. Is an example of a type 4 hypersensitivity reaction
B. Occurs after IgE antibody production in response to antigen exposure
C. Anaphylactic and anaphylactoid reactions require prior antigen exposure
D. Is most commonly caused by beta-lactam antibiotics
E. Mast cell tryptase is raised in anaphylactic but not anaphylactoid reactions

47. During the physiological changes at birth:
A. Pulmonary vascular resistance decreases slowly
B. The foramen ovale closes within hours to days
C. The ductus venosus closes due to reversal of the intracardiac shunt
D. The absence of placental circulation reduces blood flow into the IVC
E. The ductus arteriosus functionally closes within 96 hours

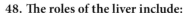

48. The roles of the liver include:
- A. Storage of vitamins D, E, K and A
- B. Synthesis of lipoproteins
- C. Degradation of C-reactive protein
- D. Gluconeogenesis
- E. Production of haptoglobins

49. The following decrease lower oesophageal sphincter (LOS) tone:
- A. Swallowing
- B. Glycopyrrolate
- C. Neostigmine
- D. Suxamethonium
- E. Morphine

50. Basal metabolic rate:
- A. Is defined as the heat production in a subject in a state of mental and physical rest in a comfortable environment 12 hours after a meal
- B. Between genders is the same when lean body mass is used as an index of comparison
- C. Typically declines at a rate of 2% per decade throughout adult life
- D. Is decreased during starvation
- E. Is increased by about 40% above normal in pregnancy

51. Within the mediastinum:
- A. Visceral pleura is sensitive to touch and pressure
- B. The anterior part contains no major blood vessels
- C. The inferior limit is the base of the heart
- D. Lymphatic tissue is present throughout all areas
- E. The division between the superior and inferior parts is a plane from the angle of Louis to the body of the sixth thoracic vertebrae

52. The following statements about the femoral triangle are correct:
- A. The femoral sheath lies next to the triangle
- B. Its superior border is the inguinal ligament
- C. Its apex lies inferiorly
- D. It contains some of the inguinal lymph nodes
- E. The abductor magnus muscle forms the medial border

53. When interpreting a chest X-ray:
- A. A posterior-anterior film magnifies the cardiac outline
- B. In an adequate inspiratory effort the right hemidiaphragm should lie below the anterior end of the sixth rib
- C. The right hilum lies at the same level as the horizontal fissure
- D. The aortic shadow should be less than 4 cm
- E. The right hilum lies 1 cm higher than the left hilum

54. For the anterior abdominal wall:
A. Innervation is provided by the posterior rami of the T7-T11 intercostal nerves
B. The internal oblique is the largest of the muscles making up the abdominal wall
C. The lower intercostal nerves travel in a plane between the external and internal oblique muscles
D. The ilioinguinal nerve supplies sensation to the skin of the upper thigh, base of penis and scrotum
E. Sensation to the gluteal region is partly supplied by the iliohypogastric nerve

55. The following statements are correct:
A. Occlusion of the anterior spinal artery will cause loss of vibration sensation
B. The anterior spinal artery is formed from a branch of the internal carotid artery
C. The posterior spinal arteries arise from the posterior inferior cerebellar arteries
D. The posterior spinal artery lies in the anterior median sulcus of the spinal cord
E. The great anterior radicular artery of Adamkiewicz supplies the upper third of the spinal cord

56. During glycolysis:
A. One pyruvate molecule is produced for every glucose molecule
B. Reactions occur primarily in the mitochondria
C. The net gain is four ATP molecules for every glucose molecule
D. Four CO_2 molecules are produced
E. No oxygen molecules are utilized

57. Sympathetic stimulation causes:
A. Increased sphincter tone
B. Bladder relaxation
C. Eyelid retraction
D. Miosis
E. Pulmonary vasoconstriction

58. The following statements are correct:
A. The pressure exerted on a capillary wall by the column of blood within it is the capillary hydrostatic pressure
B. Capillary oncotic pressure encourages the movement of water molecules out of the capillary
C. Interstitial oncotic pressure is normally 28 mmHg
D. Interstitial hydrostatic pressure is the pressure exerted on the capillary by the fluid in the interstitium, is normally 28 mmHg
E. Capillary hydrostatic pressure is kept constant along its length by autoregulation

59. Cortisol:
A. Is synthesized from 11-deoxycortisol in the zona glomerulosa
B. Causes hypertension
C. Increases glucose uptake by muscle
D. Delays foetal lung development
E. Acts by binding to a receptor on the membrane of its target cell

60. Nitric oxide:

A. Is produced by NO synthase in skeletal muscle from L-arginine
B. Activates guanylate cyclase
C. Production results in cGMP formed from guanosine triphosphate
D. Promotes smooth muscle contraction
E. Promotes platelet aggregation and adhesion

1A: False
1B: False
1C: False
1D: False
1E: False
Atracurium belongs to the benzylisoquinolinium group of non-depolarizing neuromuscular blocking agents. These compounds are composed of two quaternary amine groups joined by a central chain of methyl groups and are broken down in the plasma. Atracurium is a benzylisoquinolinium ester with four chiral molecules. This results in a preparation containing a mixture of 10 stereoisomers.

The atracurium molecule is metabolized by Hofmann degradation (60%) and ester hydrolysis (40%). Hofmann degradation occurs by cleavage of the link between the central chain and quaternary amine group, releasing laudanosine and a quaternary monoacrylate. This process occurs spontaneously in the plasma at physiological pH and temperature. Laudanosine is an inactive metabolite and is cleared from the plasma by the liver. Ester hydrolysis (of the ester bonds in the central methyl chain) occurs in the presence of non-specific esters in the plasma, producing laudanosine, a quaternary alcohol and a quaternary acid. These metabolites have insignificant neuromuscular blocking activity.

The metabolism of atracurium is therefore independent of liver and renal function, which renders it favourable for use as an infusion and in critically ill patients.

Further reading

Appiah-Ankam J, Hunter JH. Pharmacology of neuromuscular blocking drugs. *Contin Educ Anaesth Crit Care Pain*. 2004; 4(1): 2–7.

Peck TE, Hill S. *Pharmacology for Anaesthesia and Intensive Care*. 3rd ed. Cambridge: Cambridge University Press; 2008.

2A: True
2B: False
2C: False
2D: False
2E: False
Warfarin is a synthetic coumarin derivative, which is used in the prophylaxis and treatment of venous thromboembolism and to prevent thrombosis in high-risk patients (such as patients with atrial fibrillation or prosthetic valve replacements).

It acts by inhibiting the activation of vitamin K-dependent clotting factors (factors II, VII, IX and X). The activation of clotting factor precursors involves carboxylation of the glutamic acid residues on the factors and the oxidation of vitamin K to vitamin K 2,3-epoxide. Vitamin K 2,3-epoxide is reduced to vitamin K in the liver. Warfarin inhibits the reduction of vitamin K 2,3-epoxide in the liver resulting in the depletion of vitamin K-dependent clotting factors.

Warfarin is readily absorbed from the gastrointestinal tract and has a high oral bioavailability of near 100%, with peak plasma concentration occurring within an hour of ingestion. However, clinical effect is not seen until the clotting factors become depleted, with peak effect at 36 to 72 hours. Warfarin is very highly protein-bound (near 99%) to albumin in the plasma, and has a low volume of distribution. The compound is extensively metabolized in the liver by the cytochrome P450 enzymes (predominantly CYP 2C9) and excreted in the bile and urine.

The main side effect of warfarin is bleeding. Warfarin crosses the placenta with teratogenic effects and is contraindicated in both pregnancy and breastfeeding. Warfarin may cause gastrointestinal upset and hypersensitivity reactions.

Warfarin has a number of important drug interactions:

- Competition for protein binding sites (e.g. NSAIDs, hypoglycaemic agents, amiodarone), increasing free fraction of unbound warfarin and potentiating anticoagulant effects
- Interaction with metabolizing enzymes
  - Enzyme induction (e.g. rifampicin), reducing the effects of warfarin
  - Inhibition (e.g. erythromycin), increasing the effects of warfarin
- Co-administration of antihaemostatic agents (e.g. heparin, aspirin, clopidogrel), increasing the risk of major haemorrhage

Further reading

Oranmore-Brown C, Griffiths R. Anticoagulants and the perioperative period. *Contin Educ Anaesth Crit Care Pain.* 2006; 6(4): 156–159.

3A: True
3B: False
3C: False
3D: True
3E: True

Gamma-amino butyric acid (GABA) is the main inhibitory neurotransmitter in the central nervous system (CNS) and has two major receptor subtypes to which GABA binds (GABA$_A$ and GABA$_B$).

The GABA$_A$ receptor is a ligand-gated chloride ion channel composed of five subunits (2 α, β, γ and δ) surrounding a central ion channel. GABA binds and activates the GABA$_A$ receptor, increasing the frequency of opening of the channel, increasing chloride conductance and hyperpolarizing the neuronal membrane. Benzodiazepine drugs act by binding the α-subunit of the activated receptor complex, locking the receptor in an open configuration and potentiating the affinity of GABA for the receptor. The GABA$_A$ receptor is predominantly post-synaptic throughout the CNS. The GABA$_A$ receptor is further sub-classified according to its α-subunit into BZ1 and BZ2 receptors. The BZ1 subtype is present in the spinal cord and cerebellum and is responsible for anxiolysis and anterograde amnesic effects. The BZ2 subtype is present in the spinal cord, hippocampus and cortex, with sedative and anticonvulsant effects.

The GABA$_B$ receptor is a G-protein-coupled metabotropic receptor that, when stimulated, increases potassium conductance, hyperpolarizing the membrane and reducing action potential propagation. It is both a pre- and post-synaptic receptor present in the brain and dorsal horn of the spinal cord. Baclofen acts purely on the GABA$_B$ receptor to reduce spasticity.

Further reading

E-Learning Anaesthesia, Hill, S. 07c_17_01 Benzodiazepines and sedative drugs. [Online] Available from http://portal.e-lfh.org.uk.

Weir CJ. The molecular mechanisms of general anaesthesia: dissecting the GABA$_A$ receptor. *Contin Educ Anaesth Crit Care Pain.* 2006; 6(2): 49–53.

4A: False
4B: False
4C: True
4D: False
4E: True

Enzymes are biological catalysts that allow reactions to occur without themselves being altered. The relationship between the rate of enzyme and substrate reactions are described as Michaelis-Menton kinetics. The Michaelis constant (K$_m$) for an enzyme is the concentration of substrate at which the velocity of the reaction (v) is 50% its maximum (V$_{max}$). For example, hepatic enzymes with a high Michaelis constant have a high capacity for drug metabolism.

Many drugs act by altering enzyme function. Positive allosteric modulation of an enzyme by a drug may be either direct or indirect. Direct positive allosteric modulation occurs when the rate of the enzyme reaction and the affinity for its substrate are increased directly (e.g. insulin acting on tyrosine kinase). Indirect positive allosteric modulation occurs where the drug acts through a series of reactions to modulate the enzyme's activity (e.g. adrenaline is an indirect positive allosteric modulator of adenylyl cyclase by acting at the β-adrenoceptor).

Exposure to certain drugs increases hepatic cytochrome P450 enzyme activity (enzyme induction). When another drug is administered that is metabolized by these enzymes, a higher dose is required to have an equal therapeutic effect. Examples of enzyme inducers are: phenytoin, carbamazepine, barbiturates, rifampicin, alcohol and sulphonylureas (remembered by the acronym PC BRAS).

Further reading

Neal MJ. *Medical Pharmacology at a Glance.* 6th ed. Oxford: Wiley-Blackwell; 2009.

Peck TE, Hill S. *Pharmacology for Anaesthesia and Intensive Care.* 3rd ed. Cambridge: Cambridge University Press; 2008.

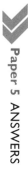

5A: True
5B: False
5C: True
5D: True
5E: True

Furosemide is a weak organic acid. The kidneys clear 85% of furosemide; half of this is metabolized and the other half is actively secreted in an unchanged form in the proximal tubules. It is highly protein-bound (>98%) and only a small fraction is filtered through the glomerulus. The presence of another highly protein-bound drug, such as warfarin, reduces furosemide's secretion and its diuretic effect. Its elimination half-life is 1.5–2 hours in healthy individuals but this is prolonged in renal failure. The site of action is at the sodium-chloride-potassium co-transporters at the intraluminal side of the ascending limb of the loop of Henle.

Further reading

Ho KM, Power BM. Benefits and risks of furosemide in acute kidney injury. *Anaesthesia*. 2010; 65: 283–293.

6A: True
6B: False
6C: False
6D: True
6E: True

Vasopressin is also known as antidiuretic hormone (ADH). It is responsible for regulating plasma osmolality and volume. It acts as a neurotransmitter in the brain controlling circadian rhythm, thermoregulation and adrenocorticotrophic hormone (ACTH) release. It is a nonapeptide and is synthesized in the paraventricular and supraoptic nuclei of the posterior hypothalamus. Vasopressin is metabolized by vasopressinases in the liver and kidney and has a half-life of 10–35 minutes. Desmopressin is a synthetic analogue of arginine vasopressin; it has 10 times the antidiuretic action of vasopressin but 1500 times less vasoconstrictor action.

Further reading

Sharman A, Low J. Vasopressin and its role in critical care. *Contin Educ Anaesth Crit Care Pain*. 2008; 8(4): 134–137.

7A: True
7B: True
7C: False
7D: True
7E: False

Gelofusine is a colloid solution containing gelatin 40 g, sodium 154 mmol·L^{-1}, chloride 124 mmol·L^{-1} and small amounts of potassium, calcium and magnesium. Gelatins are used for plasma replacement and cause a rapid increase in plasma

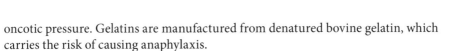

oncotic pressure. Gelatins are manufactured from denatured bovine gelatin, which carries the risk of causing anaphylaxis.

Sodium bicarbonate of 8.4% contains sodium 1000 mmol·L^{-1} and bicarbonate 1000 mmol·L^{-1} and is used in the treatment of profound metabolic acidosis. This solution has an osmolarity of 2000 mOsm·L^{-1}, thus is highly irritant to tissues if extravasated. For this reason it is often administered via a central vein. Complications are hypernatraemia, hyperosmolar syndromes and metabolic alkalosis.

Human albumin solution of 20% (20% HAS) contains albumin 200 g·L^{-1}, sodium 50–120 mmol·L^{-1}, chloride <40 mmol·L^{-1} and potassium <10 mmol·L^{-1}. Albumin is used for plasma volume expansion in haemorrhage and burns and to correct hypoalbuminaemia in critically ill patients. It is also available as a 4.5, 5 and 25% human albumin solution. Human albumin solutions carry a risk of circulatory overload, allergic reactions and aluminium toxicity.

Sodium chloride of 0.9% contains sodium 154 mmol·L^{-1} and chloride 154 mmol·L^{-1}. It is used as a maintenance and resuscitation fluid; however, its chloride content is significantly higher than that found in the plasma and may cause hyperchloraemic acidosis in excess.

Hartmann's solution contains sodium 131 mmol·L^{-1}, chloride 111 mmol·L^{-1}, potassium 5 mmol·L^{-1}, calcium 2 mmol·L^{-1} and lactate 29 mmol·L^{-1}. It is used as a maintenance or resuscitation IV fluid, and the reduced chloride concentration prevents hyperchloraemic acidosis from occurring. The lactate is metabolized in the liver to bicarbonate and glycogen; however, this may be depressed in states of hypoxia and liver dysfunction.

Further reading

Peck TE, Hill S. *Pharmacology for Anaesthesia and Intensive Care*. 3rd ed. Cambridge: Cambridge University Press; 2008.

Sasada M, Smith, S. *Drugs in Anaesthesia and Intensive Care*. 3rd ed. Oxford: Oxford University Press; 2003.

8A: False
8B: True
8C: False
8D: False
8E: True

Doxapram is used as a respiratory stimulant in patients with acute-on-chronic respiratory failure and postoperative respiratory depression. It may also be used in the treatment of laryngospasm and postoperative shivering. The drug acts primarily by stimulating the peripheral chemoreceptors and has a secondary direct action on the respiratory centre. Doxapram is only available in a parenteral preparation and acts quickly following an intravenous bolus dose of 1 mg·kg^{-1}. It has an onset of action of 20 seconds, peaks at 2 minutes and has a duration of action of 12 minutes.

Doxapram causes an increase in minute volume by increasing the tidal volume and, at higher doses, the respiratory rate. The CO_2 vs minute volume response curve is moved to the left. Other effects of doxapram are restlessness, dizziness and hallucinations alongside increased cardiac output due to an increase in the stroke volume.

Further reading

Greenstone M, Lasserson TJ. Doxapram for ventilatory failure due to exacerbations of chronic obstructive pulmonary disease. *Cochrane Database Syst Rev.* 2003; 1: CD000223.

9A: True
9B: False
9C: True
9D: False
9E: True
Dexmedetomidine is a sedative medication used in anaesthetics and intensive care. It is unusual as it causes sedation without respiratory depression. Like clonidine, it is an agonist at the α_2 adrenergic receptor. It produces a state of rousable sedation where patients can be responsive to verbal commands but then go back to sleep. It is thought that it produces a state more akin to natural sleep than the GABA-ergic hypnotics such as propofol and the benzodiazepines. Dexmedetomidine will cause bradycardia, particularly if given as a large bolus dose. It is therefore given as an infusion but has a slow onset of action where peak effects occur 10 minutes after peak plasma levels. The offset of action is also variable and context-sensitive. It is licensed for use as a sedative in critical care and is also used in general anaesthesia, where it has MAC and opioid sparing effects.

Further reading

Sleigh J. All hands on dex. *Anaesthesia.* 2012; 67: 1193–1197.

10A: True
10B: False
10C: False
10D: True
10E: False
Methadone is a synthetic opioid. It is a racemic mixture with two enantiomers, *R*-methadone and *S*-methadone. *R*-methadone is a potent μ- and δ-opioid agonist. The enantiomer *S*-methadone is inactive at the opioid receptors but it is an NMDA receptor antagonist. Partial μ-opioid agonists include tramadol, tapentadol and buprenorphine.

Methadone has an oral bioavailability of around 85%. It is highly protein-bound but mainly to α_1 acid glycoprotein. It is metabolized in the liver by the cytochrome P450 enzyme system. The metabolites are inactive and mainly excreted in the faeces. It has a long elimination phase and analgesic effect lasts for 8–12 hours. There is a risk of accumulation with repeated dosing.

Further reading

Gourlay GK, Wilson PR, Glynn CJ. Pharmacodynamics and pharmacokinetics of methadone during the perioperative period. *Anesthesiology*. 1982; 57: 458–467.

11A: False
11B: True
11C: True
11D: False
11E: False

Paracetamol, or acetaminophen, is an acetanilide. It inhibits the cyclo-oxygenase isoenzymes *COX-1* and *COX-2*. It is readily absorbed from the small bowel and does not undergo first-pass metabolism so has good oral bioavailability. Paracetamol when given rectally has a slower and less predictable rate of absorption. Paracetamol easily crosses the blood–brain barrier and the placenta as it is non-ionized at physiological pH. It is easily removed by haemodialysis.

Further reading

Oscier CD, Milner QJW. Peri-operative use of paracetamol. *Anaesthesia*. 2009; 64: 65–72.

12A: False
12B: True
12C: True
12D: False
12E: True

The volume of distribution (V_D) is a theoretical value that explains how much of a drug is distributed from the plasma to the rest of the body after oral or intravenous dosing. It is not a true physiological value. It is dependent on factors such as the lipid solubility, degree of ionization and protein binding of the drug. Highly lipid drugs such as propofol will have a high volume of distribution as they dissolve in the adipose tissue in the body (e.g. propofol). Drugs that are highly protein-bound will stay mainly in the plasma and have a low V_D (e.g. warfarin with a V_D of 8 litres). Patient factors such as changes in the size of various body compartments will affect the V_D. It is found that the V_D increases with age and in liver and renal failure.

Further reading

Roberts F, Freshwater-Turner D. Pharmacokinetics and anaesthesia. *Contin Educ Anaesth Crit Care Pain*. 2007; 7(1): 25–29.

13A: False
13B: True
13C: False
13D: False
13E: True

Local anaesthetic agents act by blocking voltage-gated sodium channels on neuronal membranes. They diffuse across the neuronal membrane in the unionized form but bind in their ionized form to the inside of the sodium channel preventing depolarization by blocking sodium conductance.

Local anaesthetics exert a greater effect on open sodium channels, as they are also able to diffuse through the open channel to access the inside.

Local anaesthetic agents consist of an aromatic group and a hydrophilic group, joined by either an ester or amide linkage. They are weak bases and exist predominantly in ionized form at physiological pH, as their pKa is above 7.4. pKa is closely related to their onset of action, as a lower pKa means more is available in a unionized form and therefore able to cross the cell membrane. This results in a faster onset of action.

Duration of action is related to degree of protein binding of the drug; those with greater protein binding having a longer duration of action.

Bupivacaine is a commonly used amide local anaesthetic agent. It has a pKa of 8.1, leading to its relatively slow onset of action; only 15% is unionized at physiological pH. It does, however, have a long duration of action, as it is 95% protein-bound. It exists as two isomers: *R*- and *S*-bupivacaine. The *S*-enantiomer is less cardiotoxic and is available as the enantiopure preparation levobupivacaine.

Further reading

Peck TE, Hill SA, Williams M. *Pharmacology for Anaesthesia and Intensive Care.* 3rd ed. Cambridge: Cambridge University Press; 2008.

Smith S, Scarth E, Sasada M. *Drugs in Anaesthesia and Intensive Care.* 4th ed. Oxford: Oxford University Press; 2011. p. 40–41.

14A: False
14B: False
14C: True
14D: True
14E: False

Drugs used to reduce plasma glucose level are used in the treatment of type II diabetes mellitus. They can be classified as those that stimulate insulin secretion, and those that increase peripheral sensitivity to circulating insulin.

Drugs that increase insulin secretion

These include sulphonylureas and meglitinides (metiglinide and repaglinide).

Sulphonylureas, such as glibenclamaide and gliclazide, are commonly used in the treatment of type II diabetes mellitus, where pancreatic β-cell function still remains. They are insulin secretagogues, which act to increase displacement of insulin from pancreatic β-cells. They also decrease glucagon secretion and peripheral insulin resistance, and lead to hyperplasia of the pancreatic β-cells.

They exist as two generations of drugs. Second-generation drugs (gliclazide, glibenclamide) are safer to use in combination with anionic drugs such as

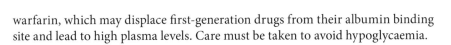

warfarin, which may displace first-generation drugs from their albumin binding site and lead to high plasma levels. Care must be taken to avoid hypoglycaemia.

Drugs that increase peripheral insulin sensitivity

Biguanides such as metformin act by increasing peripheral insulin sensitivity and therefore increase glucose uptake into cells, reducing plasma glucose concentration. In addition, they prevent production of glucose from hepatic and renal gluconeogenesis. Thiazolidinediones (e.g. rosiglitazone, pioglitazone) also increase peripheral insulin sensitivity by gene regulation.

Further reading

Peck TE, Hill SA, Williams M. *Pharmacology for Anaesthesia and Intensive Care.*
3rd ed. Cambridge: Cambridge University Press; 2008.

15A: True
15B: True
15C: True
15D: False
15E: True

A prodrug is a drug that has no inherent activity before metabolism but following metabolism in the body is converted into an active compound. This can be used to overcome problems with administration of the active drug, for example, a more lipid soluble prodrug with better absorption and diffusion across cell membranes can be metabolized to a more water-soluble compound once at the target site.

It can also be used to bypass metabolism of the active drug. For example, levodopa (*L*-DOPA) is the amino acid precursor of dopamine. It is used in the treatment of Parkinson's disease. Dopamine is unable to cross the blood–brain barrier but *L*-DOPA can, where it is converted into dopamine to have its action.

Examples of prodrugs are:

- Diamorphine: metabolized to 6-monoacylmorphine
- Enalapril: metabolized to enaloprilat
- Parecoxib: metabolized to valdecoxib
- Terlipressin: metabolized to vasopressin
- Omeprazole: metabolized to sulphenamide
- Carbimazole: metabolized to methimazole

Further reading

Peck TE, Hill SA, Williams M. *Pharmacology for Anaesthesia and Intensive Care.*
3rd ed. Cambridge: Cambridge University Press; 2008.

Smith T, Pinnock C, Lin T (Ed). *Fundamentals of Anaesthesia.* 3rd ed. Cambridge:
Cambridge University Press; 2009.

Paper 5 ANSWERS

16A: True
16B: True
16C: False
16D: True
16E: True

Transdermal drug delivery is commonly used, for instance, as fentanyl or nicotine patches. A number of specific pharmacokinetic properties are required for drugs to be able to have their effect via the transdermal route.

Advantages of the transdermal route are that it avoids first-pass metabolism in the liver, provides a constant steady-state supply of drug, avoiding large changes in plasma drug concentration and is thought to have better patient acceptability and compliance.

The main barrier to transdermal drug absorption is the stratum corneum of the skin epidermis, which must be passed before drugs can reach the dermis, where the large capillary bed confers rapid absorption into the systemic circulation. The stratum corneum contains only 20% water and is highly hydrophobic and lipophilic. Therefore, the ideal drugs for this route of delivery are small, lipophilic molecules.

The variability in thickness of stratum corneum, skin hydration, temperature as well as ethnicity and underlying skin conditions all contribute to inter-patient variability in drug absorption from transdermal drug delivery. In addition, a delay period occurs between application of the first patch or delivery system and effective plasma concentration for the drug, which may take several days.

Drugs currently available as transdermal preparations include fentanyl and buprenorphine, used in chronic pain, nicotine replacement patches and nitrates, as well as clonidine and the hormone replacement of oestrogen and testosterone.

Further reading

Margetts L, Sawyer R. Transdermal drug delivery: principles and opioid therapy. *Contin Educ Anaes Crit Care Pain.* 2007; 7(5): 171–176.

17A: True
17B: True
17C: False
17D: False
17E: True

Carbimazole is a thyroid peroxidase inhibitor and also prevents oxidation of iodide, preventing the synthesis of thyroid hormone precursors. It is a prodrug, converted in the liver to its active form, methimazole, and is used in the treatment of hyperthyroidism. It has good oral bioavailability and exhibits minimal protein binding, and is metabolized within the thyroid gland itself. Carbimazole causes rashes and itching as side effects and can rarely cause agranulocytosis; however, to a lesser extent than propylthiouracil, another drug used in the treatment of hyperthyroidism. Carbimazole does cross the placenta, which can cause problems with foetal thyroid hormone synthesis and foetal hypothyroidism. It is, however, safe for use in breastfeeding.

Further reading

Farling PA. Thyroid disease. *Brit J Anaesth.* 2000; 85(1): 15–28.

18A: False
18B: True
18C: False
18D: True
18E: False
Etomidate is a carboxylated imidazole derivative, used predominantly for induction of general anaesthesia, but also preoperatively for patients with Cushing's syndrome. It contains one chiral centre resulting in *R*- and *S*-optical isomers, of which only the *R*-form is physiologically active. It acts to enhance the effect of the inhibitory neurotransmitter GABA at the $GABA_A$ receptor, by binding to the general anaesthetic modulatory site on the β-subunit, where the *R*-isomer has over 10 times the activity of the *S*-isomer.

Etomidate is a weak base with a pKa of 4.2 and is therefore predominantly unionized at physiological pH. It is rapidly distributed to muscle and then to fat and has a volume of distribution of 4.5 L·kg^{-1}. Etomidate is metabolized by non-specific hepatic esterases and possibly plasma cholinesterase but may have an inhibitory effect on the latter. It is predominantly excreted in the urine, 2–3% unchanged, and the remainder is excreted in the bile.

It is relatively cardiostable, producing less reduction in systemic vascular resistance and minimal reduction in cardiac contractility than other intravenous anaesthetic agents. It does not impair the baroreceptor or sympathetic reflexes and blood pressure is relatively well maintained. Similarly to other intravenous agents, it causes a dose-dependent reduction in respiratory rate and tidal volume. It inhibits steroidogenesis by inhibition of adrenal 11-β and 17-α hydroxylase. Up to 15% of patients receiving etomidate experience postoperative nausea and vomiting. It can cause excitatory movements on induction as well as generalized epileptiform EEG activity but reduces intracranial pressure, cerebral blood flow and cerebral metabolic requirement for oxygen.

Further reading

Forman SA. Clinical and molecular pharmacology of etomidate. *Anesthesiology.* 2011; 114(3): 695–707.

Weir CJ. The molecular mechanisms of general anaesthesia: dissecting the $GABA_A$ receptor. *Contin Educ Anaesth Crit Care Pain.* 2006; 6(2): 49–53.

19A: True
19B: False
19C: True
19D: True
19E: False

The placenta is a complex organ that acts as the interface between foetal and maternal circulations. It develops from eroding blastocyst cells invading the decidua until multiple villi are surrounded by maternal blood. There are many factors affecting transfer of drugs and other substances across the placenta into the foetal circulation. As most drugs cross by passive diffusion, these factors are similar to those affecting diffusion across any semipermeable lipid bilayer, namely, molecular size (Graham's law), lipid solubility, pKa and its effect on ionization, and blood flow to the organ.

Factors affecting the transfer of drugs across the placenta are important when considering the safety of maternal drug administration in pregnancy. Highly lipid-soluble drugs, such as opiates and induction agents, readily cross the placenta and can be detected within the foetal circulation. Similarly, drugs that are highly unionized at physiological pH favour placental transfer. In addition, foetal acid-base abnormalities can influence placental-to-foetal transfer and can lead to trapping of drugs, for example, basic drugs such as local anaesthetics become trapped in the foetus, which is acidotic as they become increasingly ionized and therefore unable to transfer back to the maternal circulation. Large ionized molecules, such as muscle relaxants, are not able to cross the placenta and similarly ionized quaternary ammonium compounds such as neostigmine undergo limited placental transfer.

Further reading

Chestnut DH. *Obstetric Anaesthesia Principles and Practice*. 3rd ed. Philadelphia: Elsevier Mosby; 2004. Chapter 4, p. 49–65.

Peck TE, Hill SA, Williams M. *Pharmacology for Anaesthesia and Intensive Care*. 3rd ed. Cambridge: Cambridge University Press; 2008. Chapter 1, p. 1–7.

20A: False
20B: False
20C: True
20D: False
20E: True

Opioid receptors are G-protein-coupled receptors that act via a second messenger system. There are four subtypes of opioid receptor, classified according to their endogenous ligands and location.

- μ-opioid (or MOP) receptors are located throughout the central nervous system, including within the dorsal horns of the spinal cord and within the periaqueductal grey of the midbrain. MOP agonists confer analgesic properties but are also associated with some unwanted side effects, such as respiratory depression.
- κ-opioid (or KOP) receptors are located within primary cells of the nucleus raphe magnus (NRM), and are not associated with respiratory depression but can have anti-opioid effects, limiting the analgesia achieved by MOP agonists.
- δ-opioid (or DOP) receptors are the least widely distributed, found within the olfactory bulb, cerebral cortex, nucleus accumbens and caudate putamen. They are responsible for some of the analgesic effects of opioids but also cause constipation due to reduced gastric motility, as well as respiratory depression.

The most recently classified opioid receptor is the nociception-opioid (or NOP) receptor, which is thought to be responsible for opioid tolerance. In fact, NOP agonists lead to sensitization to nociceptive stimuli, whereas antagonists at the NOP receptor are thought to be useful for long lasting analgesia.

Further reading

McDonald J, Lambert DG. Opioid receptors. *Contin Educ Anaesth Crit Care Pain.* 2005; 5(1): 22–25.

Smith S, Scarth E, Sasada M. *Drugs in Anaesthesia and Intensive Care.* 4th ed. Oxford: Oxford University Press; 2011. p. 136–149.

21A: False
21B: True
21C: False
21D: False
21E: False
Core temperature is the temperature of internal organs within the body, such as the brain. Sites that can be used for measuring core body temperature are the tympanic membrane, nasopharynx, distal oesophagus, pulmonary artery, rectum and bladder.

- The tympanic membrane can be measured using the infrared probe, which is non-invasive and accurate
- The nasopharynx is easily accessible and accurate when the probe is positioned well, although cannot comfortably be used in non-anaesthetized patients
- The lower quarter of the oesophagus is accurate as it gives a reading that is not affected by respiratory gas flow
- The pulmonary artery catheter is the gold standard for core body temperature measurement; however, it is invasive and not appropriate for the majority of cases
- Rectal temperature measurement can alter in the presence of faeces and has a significant lag time
- Measurement of bladder temperature is an accurate reflection of core body temperature; however, it is invasive

Further reading

Sullivan G, Edmondson C. Heat and temperature. *Contin Educ Anaesth Crit Care Pain.* 2008; 8(3): 104–107.

22A: False
22B: False
22C: False
22D: True
22E: True
The gas laws describe the behaviour of gases by three parameters: pressure, temperature and volume.

They are calculated on the premise of an ideal gas (sometimes called 'perfect' gases), in which molecules occupy no volume and are not affected by intermolecular forces.

- Boyle's law: at a constant temperature, the volume of a given mass of gas varies inversely with absolute pressure

$$pV = k$$

- Charles' law: at a constant pressure, the volume of a given mass of gas is directly proportional to the absolute temperature

$$V = kT$$

- Gay-Lussac's law: at a constant volume, the absolute pressure of a given mass of gas is proportional to the absolute temperature

$$p = kT$$

- The combined gas law: this combines Boyle's, Charles' and Gay-Lussac's laws

$$pV/T = k$$

In all of the above
  p = pressure
  V = volume
  T = absolute temperature (Kelvin)
  k = constant

- The ideal gas law: this combines Avogadro's law (that the same volume of gases contains the same number of molecules) with the combined gas law to state

$$pV = nRT$$

where
  n = amount of substance (moles)
  R = universal gas constant (8.314 J·K^{-1}·mol^{-1})

- Dalton's law of partial pressures: in a mixture of gases, the pressure exerted by each gas is the same as that which it would exert if it alone occupied the container

$$P_{total} = P_1 + P_2 + P_3, \ldots$$

- Henry's law: at a constant temperature, the amount of gas dissolved in a liquid is proportional to the partial pressure of the gas (above the solvent) in equilibrium with the liquid

$$p_{gas} = k_H c$$

where
  p_{gas} = partial pressure of gas above liquid (atm)
  k_H = Henry's constant
  c = solubility of gas

Further reading

Davis PD, Kenny GNC. *Basic Physics and Measurement in Anaesthesia*. 5th ed. Oxford: Butterworth-Heinemann; 2003.

23A: False
23B: True
23C: False
23D: True
23E: True

Thermodilution is a mechanism of invasive monitoring that uses the Fick principle to calculate cardiac output.

The Fick principle states that the amount of substance taken up by an organ per unit time is equal to the arterial concentration minus the venous concentration of the substance, multiplied by the blood flow through the organ. This can be used to calculate flow (or cardiac output), where:

Blood flow = Rate of uptake/Arterial – Venous concentration difference

or

$$Q = (VO_2/(C_A - C_V)) \times 100$$

where
  Q = blood flow
  VO_2 = oxygen consumption
  C_A = oxygen content of arterial blood
  C_V = oxygen content of venous blood

Thermodilution uses a pulmonary artery catheter inserted into a central vein and floated through the right atrium, right ventricle and into the pulmonary artery. The catheter has multiple lumens: a proximal lumen (30 cm from the catheter tip), which opens in the right atrium and a distal lumen (3.7 cm from the catheter tip), which contains a thermistor and sits in the pulmonary artery.

Ten millilitres of ice-cold saline is injected into the proximal port in the right atrium, where it circulates through the heart into the pulmonary artery. The thermistor detects a change in temperature with time and plots a graph of temperature against time. The area under this temperature/time graph is inversely proportional to cardiac output. From this graph, the cardiac output can be calculated using the Stewart–Hamilton equation (a variation of the Fick principle).

Thermodilution measures the cardiac output of the right heart to give us a global cardiac output measurement. The accuracy of the thermodilution technique may be reduced by:

1. Cardiac shunt (altering right and left ventricular output)
2. Tricuspid or pulmonary regurgitation (underestimation of cardiac output)
3. Variation in blood temperature (e.g. cardiac bypass)
4. Positive pressure ventilation (alteration in right ventricular stroke volume on a beat to beat basis)

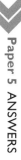

Further reading

Allsager CM, Swanevelder J. Measuring cardiac output. *Contin Educ Anaesth Crit Care Pain*. 2003; (3)1: 15–19.

24A: True
24B: True
24C: True
24D: True
24E: False

Audible sound is in the frequency range of 20 to 20 000 hertz (Hz). Ultrasound is defined as sound waves at a frequency greater than 20 000 Hz. Medical ultrasound utilizes frequencies of typically 2–10 MHz. Ultrasound is generated by the application of a voltage across a crystal, causing it to contract and relax and resulting in the generation of pressure, or sound waves. This effect of converting electrical energy into sound energy is the piezoelectric effect.

The ultrasound wave generated through the piezoelectric effect is transmitted through tissues. Where two tissues with different acoustic impedances meet (e.g. air and bone), ultrasound waves will either continue to pass through the tissue or are reflected back to the probe. The acoustic impedance of a tissue is determined by the density of the tissue and the propagation speed (the speed at which sound waves travel through it). The greater the difference in acoustic impedance between the tissues encountered, the greater the degree of reflection and the greater the intensity of the reflected wave. The reflected waves are converted to electrical signals and displayed as an image, where each wave appears as a dot on the monitor screen. The brightness of this dot reflects the intensity of the reflected wave. For example, bone reflects a large proportion of ultrasound waves and therefore appears brighter on the screen.

Further reading

Aldrich J. Basic physics of ultrasound imaging. *Crit Care Med*. 2007; 35, 5(Suppl): S131–S137.

25A: True
25B: True
25C: False
25D: False
25E: True

Understanding the functioning of a fibreoptic bundle requires an understanding of some of the principles of light.

When light travelling through one medium comes into contact with another medium, the angle at which it comes into contact with the second medium (from a 'normal' line at right angles to the medium) is known as the angle of incidence.

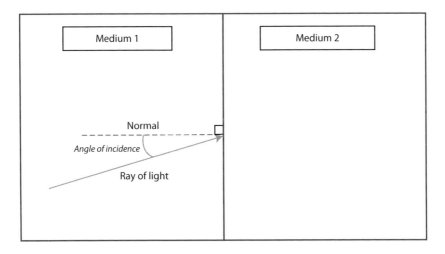

Reflection occurs when the surface the light hits is shiny. The light bounces back at the same angle as the angle of incidence, known as the angle of reflection.

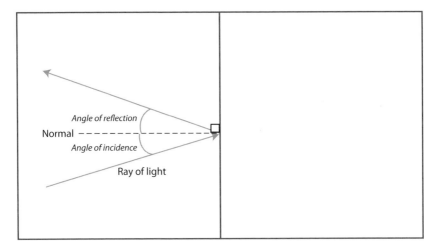

Because light travels at different speeds in different mediums, if light passes into another medium it will bend, which is known as refraction. The degree of refraction depends on the angle of incidence and the refractive index of the medium (the speed at which light travels in it compared to speed within a vacuum).

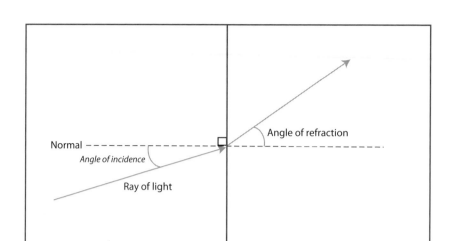

Total internal reflection occurs when the ray of light hits the junction between two mediums at an angle greater than the critical angle. This is the principle involved in optical fibres. The light is contained within the centre of the fibre and does not pass through into the outer covering, a medium with a lower refractive index.

Further reading

Berge D, Pearce A. Physics in anaesthesia: the fibreoptic intubating laryngoscope. *Update in Anaesthesia*. 2005; 19(3): 166–170.

26A: False
26B: False
26C: True
26D: False
26E: True
Nerve stimulators administer electrical stimuli to peripheral nerves and can be used to assess neuromuscular blockade. A supramaximal stimulus is applied to the nerve (commonly the ulnar or facial nerve) in a number of different patterns and the motor response may be measured in a number of ways:

● Clinically
● Electromyography
● Mechanomyography
● Acellerometry
● Piezoelectric methods

Supramaximal stimulus: a stimulus sufficient to make all the axons in a nerve discharge.

● Single twitch: a single supramaximal stimulus. Commonly >60 mA for 0.2 ms.
● Train of four: four single twitch square wave stimuli applied for 0.2 ms at 2 Hz (i.e. one every 500 ms). The ratio of the amplitude of the fourth to the first twitches is called train of four ratio and can be used to assess receptor site occupancy and suitability for reversal.

- Tetanic stimulus: supramaximal 0.2 ms stimuli applied at 50 Hz for 5 seconds. When monitoring deep neuromuscular blockade a post-tetanic count may be performed by applying 20 single twitch stimuli at 1 Hz 3 seconds after a tetanic stimulus. The result of the count is specific to the neuromuscular blocking agent used.
- Double burst stimulus: two bursts of three stimuli at 50 Hz, with 750 ms separating the two bursts. The ratio between the first twitch and the last twitch can also be used to assess adequacy of reversal.

Further reading

Davey AJ, Diba A. *Ward's Anaesthetic Equipment*. 5th ed. Philadelphia: Elsevier Saunders; 2005. Chapter 19, p. 381–383.

Plunkett E, Cross M. *Physics, Pharmacology and Physiology for Anaesthetists*. Cambridge: Cambridge University Press; 2008. Section 2, p. 69–73.

27A: True
27B: False
27C: False
27D: True
27E: True

Infrared spectrophotometry works on the principle that gases with two or more dissimilar atoms in each molecule will absorb infrared radiation at a specific wavelength to the individual gas. By selecting the infrared wavelength and understanding the components of the gas mixture, this principle can be used to measure a particular gas of interest and avoid others. Infrared radiation is emitted (commonly by a hot wire) and passed through a filter to select the frequency and wavelength required. This beam then passes through a sample chamber and is focused on a photodetector. The greater the number of carbon dioxide molecules, the greater the absorption of infrared; this is used to derive the partial pressure of carbon dioxide in the gas. Often the filters are mounted on a rotating disc, which allows simultaneous analysis of other expired gases.

Inaccuracies can result from variation in infrared source output and in the sensitivity of the photodetector. A double-beam instrument can be used, which incorporates a second beam that bypasses the sample chamber to pass through a reference chamber. This accounts for detection of changes in output, which are not caused by changes in carbon dioxide concentration.

Collision broadening occurs when carbon dioxide is in a gas mixture with nitrous oxide. When carbon dioxide and nitrous oxide molecules collide in the gas mixture, they interact to broaden the bandwidth of absorption by carbon dioxide. This can lead to a false overestimation of the partial pressure of carbon dioxide in the presence of nitrous oxide.

Further reading

Langton JA, Hutton A. Respiratory gas analysis. *Contin Educ Anaesth Crit Care Pain*. 2009; 9(1): 19–23.

28A: False
28B: False
28C: True
28D: False
28E: False

Critical temperature is the temperature above which a gas cannot be liquefied, no matter how much pressure is applied. The critical temperature of N_2O is 36.5°C and of O_2 is –119°C.

Critical pressure is the minimum pressure required to liquefy a gas at its critical temperature.

Critical volume is the volume occupied by 1 mole of a gas at its critical temperature and critical pressure.

Pseudocritical temperature refers to a mixture of gases. It is the temperature at which a gas mixture will separate into its constituents (the Poynting effect). For Entonox™, this is –5.5°C in a cylinder, 30°C in a pipeline.

Avogadro's hypothesis states that equal volumes of gases (at standard temperature and pressure, STP) contain equal numbers of molecules. One mole of any gas occupies 22.4 litres at STP and contains 6.02×10^{23} molecules.

Further reading

Davis PD. *Basic Physics and Measurement in Anaesthesia*. 5th ed. Oxford: Butterworth-Heinemann; 2003.

Smith T, Pinnock C, Lin T. *Fundamentals of Anaesthesia*. 3rd ed. Cambridge: Cambridge University Press; 2009. p. 253–258.

29A: True
29B: True
29C: True
29D: True
29E: False

When a substance changes from liquid to gas, or from solid to liquid, latent heat energy is required to break the bonds holding the molecules together. Energy is released (from stored potential energy in the bonds in the substance) to the environment. As a substance vaporizes, the remaining liquid will cool due to loss of heat energy.

Latent heat of vaporization is the energy required to change a substance from liquid to gas without changing its temperature.

Latent heat of fusion is the energy required to change a substance from solid to liquid without changing its temperature.

An isobologram is a graph used to describe drug interactions.

Further reading

Smith T, Pinnock C, Lin T. *Fundamentals of Anaesthesia*. 3rd ed. Cambridge: Cambridge University Press; 2009.

30A: True
30B: False
30C: False
30D: True
30E: True
A line isolation system consists of an isolating transformer and a line isolation monitor, which produce a 'floating circuit', protecting the patient from connection to earth. The line isolation monitor alarms and disconnects if the patient circuit inadvertently connects to earth. The earth-free supply is safe; however, it is impractical for the entire theatre to be isolated as a fault in one device will shut off the entire supply to the theatre. Thus, in practice, individual electrical devices are isolated.

Further reading

Boumphrey S, Langton JA. Electrical safety in the operating theatre. *Contin Educ Anaesth Crit Care Pain*. 2003; 3(1):10–14.

Smith T, Pinnock C, Lin T. *Fundamentals of Anaesthesia*. 3rd ed. Cambridge: Cambridge University Press; 2009. p. 253–258.

31A: False
31B: False
31C: True
31D: False
31E: True
Heat loss occurs in both general and regional anaesthesia. Core body temperature drops by 0.5–1°C within the first hour mainly due to redistribution of heat from the core to the periphery. The rate of loss afterwards is 0.3°C per hour. Infusion of 1 litre of room temperature fluid can reduce core temperature by 0.5°C.

Temperature loss occurs through five main mechanisms. They are (in descending order): radiation, convection, evaporation, respiration and conduction.

- Radiation represents 40% of heat loss and relates to the Stefan–Boltzmann law.
- Convection (30%) refers to convection currents being produced by air being heated and becoming less dense and rising. This is the same process in household radiators.
- Evaporation (15%) causes heat loss through the latent heat of vaporization. This is the energy that is needed to change the state of a liquid to a gas.
- Respiration (10%) includes another source of evaporative heat loss restricted to the airways.
- Conduction (5%) involves heat transfer between two objects of different temperature.

Further reading

Sullivan G, Edmondson C. Heat and temperature. *Contin Educ Anaesth Crit Care Pain*. 2008; 8: 104–107.

32A: False
32B: False
32C: True
32D: False
32E: True

SI stands for Système International d'Unités. There are actually three types of SI units: fundamental, derived and supplementary. There are only two supplementary units: the unit of plane angle (the radian) and the unit of solid angle (the steradian). There are seven fundamental units, from which many units are derived. The seven fundamental units are: the mole, second, ampere, candela, metre, kelvin, and the kilogram (not the gram).

Further reading

Marval P. SI units and simple respiratory and cardiac mechanics. *Contin Educ Anaesth Crit Care Pain*. 2006; 6: 188–191.

33A: False
33B: True
33C: True
33D: False
33E: True

Desflurane has two characteristics that make it unsuitable for use in traditional vaporizers. Compared with other volatile anaesthetic agents, desflurane has a high saturated vapour pressure (SVP) and a low boiling point. These properties mean that a very high fresh gas flow would be needed to dilute the vapour to clinically useful concentrations and it will intermittently boil at room temperature. This means that a different type of vaporizer from the traditional variable bypass is required.

The TEC 6 desflurane vaporizer is an example of a measured flow vaporizer. The principle of this type of vaporizer is that there is a separate stream of anaesthetic vapour that is added to the fresh gas flow. The vaporizer must measure and adjust for changes in the fresh gas flow. To overcome the physical properties of desflurane, the TEC 6 vaporizer utilizes an electrically powered heating element to heat the desflurane to 39°C. This raises its SVP to 194 kPa. To provide accurate agent concentrations, the amount of agent added is proportional to the fresh gas flow. This is achieved by using a differential pressure transducer. There is a flow restriction in the fresh gas flow. Any increase in flow will produce a back pressure, which acts on the differential pressure transducer. This then acts on a variable resistor at the agent outflow to increase agent flow in-line with the fresh gas flow. Vice versa is also true.

Further reading

Boumphrey S, Marshall S. Understanding vaporizers. *Contin Educ Anaesth Crit Care Pain*. 2011; 11: 199–203.

34A: True
34B: True
34C: False
34D: False
34E: True

An electromanometer is a pressure sensing system that converts the mechanical energy into an electrical signal so it can be displayed and recorded. We commonly use this when measuring arterial blood pressure. The setup contains a cannula in continuity with arterial blood stream and a fluid filled catheter that has a flexible diaphragm on one end that is connected to a microprocessor. Each setup will have a resonant frequency that is unique to it. This resonant or natural frequency is dependent on the radius of the catheter, the length of the catheter, the stiffness of the diaphragm and the density of the fluid in the system. When there is a change in the pressure in the system there is a tendency for the output signal to oscillate about the new pressure level.

Damping is the tendency to reduce these oscillations. The same factors that influence the natural frequency influence the level of damping but in an inverse manner. Factors that increase damping are long, narrow catheters, stiff diaphragms and fluids of high densities or the presence of clot or air in the catheter. In response to a stepwise change in pressure an overdamped system will have no oscillation but will take time to reach the new pressure level. An underdamped system will reach that level quicker but will overshoot and oscillate about the new pressure level.

An undamped system has a damping ratio of 0, optimally damped 0.66 and critically damped 1.

Further reading

Dolenska S. *Basic Science for Anaesthetists*. Cambridge: Cambridge University Press; 2006.

35A: True
35B: True
35C: True
35D: True
35E: False

The supply chain of medical gases from storage device to patient follows a stepwise decrease in pressure. Different units are used to define the pressure at various stages, dependent on the magnitude of that pressure. Bar is used to describe high pressures, psi for moderate, mmHg for atmospheric pressures and cmH_2O for very low pressures.

An oxygen cylinder will have a pressure of 137 bar (or 137×1000 cmH_2O). Nitrous oxide cylinders have a pressure of around 55 bar (or 55×0.1 MPa). Carbon dioxide cylinders also have this pressure but are no longer used clinically. The gas pipeline has a pressure of 4 bar (or 750 mmHg $\times$ 4). The back bar on an anesthetic machine has a relief valve set at 0.34 bar (or 34 kPa or 340 cmH_2O). The adjustable pressure limiting (or APL) valve is set to blow off at 50–60 cmH_2O or 5–6 kPa.

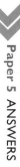

Further reading

Dolenska S. *Basic Science for Anaesthetists*. Cambridge: Cambridge University Press; 2006.

36A: False
36B: True
36C: False
36D: False
36E: False

Clinical studies can be broadly grouped into retrospective or prospective studies. Retrospective studies look backward at a population that has been exposed to a risk or preventative factor and compare that to some outcome that has been proposed. By comparison, prospective studies look forward in time at a patient population and compare how their outcome is affected either by some intervention or change in risk exposure. Examples of retrospective studies include cross-sectional studies, surveys and case-control studies. Prospective studies include observational cohort studies, randomized or non-randomized controlled trials.

Retrospective trials are relatively cheap to run and can involve using data already collected from databases or registers. They are useful when investigating rare diseases where the number of patients would be too low to include in a prospective study. Also if the lag time between risk exposure and outcome is very long, for example, mesothelioma, then a prospective study would have to run for years to find any conclusions. The drawbacks include recall bias from surveys, interviews or data collection from notes. There is also the inability to randomize patients to an exposure and control group. In the case-control study each case is matched to an ideal control but this has inherent problems and is a source of potential bias.

Further reading

Lalkhen AG, McCluskey A. Statistics V: introduction to clinical trials and systematic reviews. *Contin Educ Anaesth Crit Care Pain*. 2008; 8(4): 143–146.

37A: False
37B: True
37C: False
37D: False
37E: True

The null hypothesis assumes that there is no difference in the specified variable between study groups.

When considering the results of a study with respect to the null hypothesis, the results may not always reflect the true relationship between the study groups.

A type II (β) error is a false negative. In reality there is a difference between the groups but the study has failed to find it. This is usually due to small study numbers. The null hypothesis is therefore accepted incorrectly.

A type I (α) error, or false positive, rejects the null hypothesis as a statistically significant difference is found when in reality no difference exists between the study groups. A standard *P* value of 0.05 is used, rather than 0.5, to demonstrate statistical significance and reject the null hypothesis.

The power of a study is the likelihood of the null hypothesis being correctly rejected and is calculated by 1 minus the probability of type II (β) error.

Further reading

McCluskey A, Lalkhen AG. Statistics IV: interpreting the results of statistical tests. *Contin Educ Anaesth Crit Care Pain.* 2007; 7(6): 208–212.

38A: False
38B: False
38C: False
38D: True
38E: False

A 12-lead ECG uses 10 electrodes and gives 12 views of the electrical activity in the heart. This is impractical for anaesthesia so 3 (or occasionally 5) electrodes are used. This gives 3 views of the electrical activity of the heart or 3 leads. The common placement for the ECG electrodes is the right arm, left arm and left leg (usually placed on the left side of the chest). One electrode acts as a neutral and the potential difference (PD) is measured between the remaining two.

Lead I measures the PD between the right arm and left arm; lead II between the right arm and left leg; lead III between the left arm and left leg. Lead II is best for detecting the presence of any arrhythmias as it allows the best view of P and R waves. For detecting myocardial ischaemia a different electrode position can be used.

The CM5 configuration places the right arm on the manubrium, the left arm at the position of V5 (from the 12-lead ECG configuration) and the left leg on the clavicle. Setting the monitor to Lead I will pick up 80% of ischaemia and still be good for detecting arrhythmias too.

Further reading

Al Shaikh B, Stacey S. *Essentials of Anaesthetic Equipment.* Edinburgh: Churchill Livingstone; 2007.

39A: True
39B: False
39C: True
39D: False
39E: True

There are a number of devices used in anaesthesia to measure pulmonary function. They can be used to measure lung volumes as well as gas flow. The most common are simple spirometers and peak expiratory flowmeters.

The Benedict-Roth spirometer involves a bell, which moves with the patient's breathing; recorded on a rotating drum by a pen that transmits movement of the bell. However, it is large and difficult to transport.

The vitalograph consists of a lightweight bellows, which is filled with expired gas, causing a pen to move across a constantly moving chart, producing a volume–time graph. Volumes and flow rates may be calculated from this graph.

The Wright respirometer measures tidal volumes by monitoring the movement of a vane that is rotated by the flow of gas. It does not produce an electronic output but is small and portable. It is calibrated for tidal ventilation but is inaccurate for measurement of continuous gas flow as the vane does not rotate in reverse flow.

Wright's peak flowmeter is a constant pressure-variable orifice device. The exhaled gas from the patient causes a vane to rotate, opposed by a coiled spring attached to a pointer, which registers its movement. As the vane rotates to maintain a constant pressure, it opens a slot to allow gas to escape, altering the orifice of the device. The mini-Wright peak flowmeter is a more portable, cylindrical device, which also acts on the variable orifice constant pressure principle.

The pneumotachograph is used to obtain an electrical signal proportional to flow. A gauze screen acts as a small resistance to flow, resulting in a small pressure drop across the screen. This can be transduced to an electrical display. It can rapidly demonstrate respiratory changes but as it relies on laminar flow, it can be affected by change in temperature (and therefore viscosity) of gas.

Further reading

Davey AJ, Diba A. *Ward's Anaesthetic Equipment*. 5th ed. Philadelphia: Elsevier Saunders; 2005. Chapter 4, p. 60–64.

Davis PD, Kenny GNC. *Basic Physics and Measurement in Anaesthesia*. 5th ed. Oxford: Butterworth-Heinemann; 2003. Chapter 3, p. 23–30.

40A: False
40B: False
40C: True
40D: False
40E: True

The SI unit for absorbed radiation dose is the grey (Gy), for equivalent dose it is the sievert (Sv). The becquerel (Bq) is the SI unit for radioactivity. The radiation from a chest X-ray is equivalent to 3 days background exposure, skull 11 days, abdominal 4 months, CT chest abdomen 4 years. The lifetime cancer risk from a CT chest and abdomen is 1 in 2000–2500. The exposure from fluoroscopy is not minimal. Generalization is difficult as exposure is affected by many factors. These include patient age, size and body composition. The procedure and the technique, and experience of the physician, and also the beam magnification, distance of the patient from source and screening technique also affect exposure. The accumulated annual exposure to a pain physician is equivalent to 1 CT abdomen per year.

Further reading

Taylor J, Chandramohan M, Simpson K. Radiation safety for anaesthetists. *Contin Educ Anaesth Crit Care Pain*. 2013; 13(2): 59–62.

41A: True
41B: True
41C: True
41D: False
41E: True

Magnesium is the second most abundant intracellular cation, after sodium. Normal plasma concentrations of magnesium are 0.7–1.05 mmol·L⁻¹; this level is regulated by control of gastrointestinal absorption and renal excretion. Magnesium is freely filtered at the glomerulus and then the majority is reabsorbed in the ascending loop of Henle. Usually only 1% of filtered magnesium is excreted in the urine. Magnesium is an essential cofactor in ATP-dependent processes as ATP requires magnesium chelation to be fully active. In addition, magnesium plays a role in many important physiological processes. It is a non-competitive antagonist at voltage-gated calcium channels and inhibits acetylcholine release at the neuromuscular junction, which may explain why it prolongs the duration of action of both depolarizing and non-depolarizing neuromuscular blockers.

Further reading

Parikh M, Webb ST. Cations: potassium, calcium and magnesium. *Contin Educ Anaesth Crit Care Pain.* 2012; 12(4): 195–198.

Watson VF, Vaughan RS. Magnesium and the anaesthetist. *Contin Educ Anaesth Crit Care Pain.* 2001; 1(1): 16–20.

42A: False
42B: True
42C: False
42D: True
42E: True

The sino-atrial node (SAN) has the highest rate of automaticity of the pacemaker cells and therefore determines the rate of cardiac muscle contraction. Cells of the SAN do not have a stable resting membrane potential but rather have a pacemaker potential that gradually increases towards a threshold potential of approximately –50 mV due to decreased potassium permeability and a slow inward current of calcium due to opening of voltage-gated T-type calcium channels. Once threshold potential is reached, voltage-gated L-type calcium channels open and are responsible for the influx of calcium ions that leads to depolarization. In contrast to ventricular myocytes, cells of the SAN do not have a plateau phase (phase 1 or 2) in their action potential.

Further reading

Pinnell J, Turner S, Howell S. Cardiac muscle physiology. *Contin Educ Anaesth Crit Care Pain.* 2007; 7(3): 85–88.

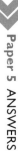

43A: False
43B: True
43C: False
43D: False
43E: False

Physiological dead space encompasses all areas of the respiratory tract that are not available for gas exchange. This includes anatomical dead space (the volume of the conducting airways) and alveolar dead space (the volume of alveoli that are not perfused). Anatomical dead space is approximately 2 ml·kg⁻¹ or 150 ml in an adult male. Physiological dead space can be calculated using the Bohr equation, whereas Fowler's method (nitrogen washout) is used to determine the volume of anatomical dead space and closing volume.

Physiological dead space is increased by factors reducing alveolar perfusion, such as hypotension or pulmonary embolism, as well as factors increasing anatomical dead space, such as standing, extending the neck or bronchodilation.

Further reading

Fletcher R, et al. The concept of dead space with special further reading to the single breath test for carbon dioxide. *Br J Anaesth.* 1981; 53(1): 77–88.

West JB. *Respiratory Physiology: The Essentials.* 8th ed. Philadelphia: Lippincott Williams & Wilkins; 2008.

44A: False
44B: False
44C: True
44D: True
44E: False

Tidal volume (V_T) is the volume of air expired in normal tidal breathing following a normal inspiration. The volume of air that can be forcibly expired following tidal expiration is known as expiratory reserve volume (ERV), and similarly the volume of air that can be inspired forcibly following normal inspiration is the inspiratory reserve volume (IRV). The sum of both the inspiratory and expiratory reserve volumes and the tidal volume is known as the vital capacity (VC). All these volumes can be measured by simple spirometry. The volume of air remaining in the lung following tidal expiration is the functional residual capacity (FRC). This includes the residual volume (RV) of the lung, which is the volume of air remaining in the lung after maximal forced expiration. The RV and any capacities that include it (total lung capacity [TLC] and FRC) cannot be measured by simple spirometry but can be determined by body plethysmography or helium dilution.

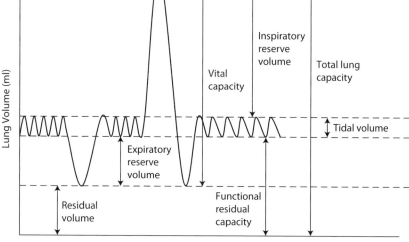

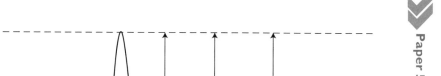

45A: False
45B: False
45C: False
45D: False
45E: False

The neuromuscular junction (NMJ) is made up of a motor nerve and a muscle cell, separated by a space called the synaptic cleft. Molecules of the neurotransmitter acetylcholine (ACh) released by the motor nerve travel across this cleft and lead to depolarization of the muscle cell by interaction with ACh receptors on the post-synaptic membrane of the muscle cell.

Each motor nerve branches into multiple terminals, each of which can innervate one neuromuscular junction. Each muscle cell takes part in only one neuromuscular junction but the muscle cells that are innervated by terminals of a particular motor neurone are together known as a motor unit.

The area of the post-synaptic membrane that forms part of the neuromuscular junction is called the motor endplate, and contains 1–10 million ACh receptors.

ACh is formed in the cytoplasm of the motor nerve axon from choline and acetyl coenzyme A in the presence of the enzyme choline acetyltransferanse. It is mostly stored in vesicles within the cytoplasm of the nerve axon and released in response to calcium influx through P-type calcium channels following a nerve impulse. 50–100 vesicles, each containing approximately 12000 molecules of ACh, are released into the synaptic cleft, where they bind to nicotinic ACh receptors on the motor endplate.

Nicotinic ACh receptors are transmembrane receptors composed of five protein subunits (two α, β, δ and ε) with a central ion channel. Binding of two ACh molecules to the α subunits causes a conformational change, opening the cation channel. Sodium influx is predominantly responsible for depolarization of the motor endplate and subsequent action potential propagation and muscle cell contraction.

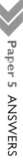

ACh is removed from the synaptic cleft by acetylcholinesterase, and the resulting choline is taken back up into the presynaptic nerve terminal and used to form further ACh.

Further reading

King JM, Hunter JM. Physiology of the neuromuscular junction. *Contin Educ Anaesth Crit Care Pain.* 2002; 2(5): 129–133.

46A: False
46B: True
46C: False
46D: False
46E: False

Hypersensitivity describes an otherwise beneficial immune response that is exaggerated or inappropriate, causing tissue damage.

Type I hypersensitivity reactions, also known as immediate hypersensitivity, are IgE-mediated reactions. Activation of B-lymphocytes by T helper cells and antigen presenting cells leads to IgE production. After initial antigen exposure antibody levels decrease but IgE remains attached to mast cells, which, on further exposure to antigen, causes them to degranulate, releasing inflammatory mediators such as histamine, leukotrienes, cytokine and platelet activating factor. The location of the antigen determines the clinical effect, which includes smooth muscle contraction, vasodilatation and increased vascular permeability. When this type of hypersensitivity reaction is widespread, it causes anaphylaxis.

- Type I hypersensitivity
  - Immediate
  - IgE mediated
- Type II hypersensitivity
  - IgM/IgG mediated
  - Complement cascade activation
  - e.g. Goodpastures syndrome, Myasthenia Gravis
- Type III hypersensitivity
  - Immune complex deposition
  - e.g. Rheumatoid arthritis, SLE
- Type IV hypersensitivity
  - Delayed
  - Cell-mediated
  - Contact/tuberculin type or granulomatous (e.g. TB)

Anaphylactoid reactions are clinically impossible to distinguish from anaphylaxis, involving airway oedema, bronchospasm and hypotension but are not mediated by IgE. They are caused by release of vasoactive mediators, direct histamine release or complement activation. They do not require previous antigen sensitization.

The most common cause of anaphylaxis in anaesthesia is neuromuscular blocking agents, with suxamethonium identified as the cause in 43% of these. The most common cause of anaphylactoid reactions is contrast media.

Investigations should be carried out following resuscitation and stabilization of the patient to determine the nature of the reaction. Initial blood tests for serum mast cell tryptase should be taken as soon as is safe to do so, and at 1 and 6–24 hours after the reaction. Tryptase is an enzyme contained mostly (99%) within mast cells. It is released by mast cell degranulation, with maximal serum concentration seen at about 1 hour. It is raised in both anaphylaxis and anaphylactoid reactions, and distinguishes them from other potential causes of the event but will not identify the causative agent. This can be determined by later investigations including skin prick testing and assays for specific IgE antibodies.

Further reading

Ryder SA, Waldmann C. Anaphylaxis. *Contin Educ Anaesth Crit Care Pain.* 2004; 4(4): 111–113.

47A: False
47B: False
47C: False
47D: True
47E: True
At birth, several changes must take place within the foetal circulation to allow the neonate to function in the extra-uterine environment. Gas exchange must now take place in the pulmonary circulation, as the placental circulation is no longer available.

After expansion of the lungs, pulmonary blood flow increases 8- to 10-fold as pulmonary vascular resistance decreases. This occurs due to both reversal of hypoxic pulmonary vasoconstriction and reflex vasodilatation mediated by pulmonary stretch receptors, as well as physical expansion of the lung.

Increased venous return to the left atrium (which previously only received 12% of cardiac output from the pulmonary circulation) and decreased venous return to the right atrium (due to removal of placental circulation and decreased flow through ductus venosus) allows the left atrial and right atrial pressures to equalize and effectively close the foramen ovale intracardiac shunt. This occurs within minutes to hours.

The ductus venosus closes passively 3–10 days after birth following the disappearance of the placental circulation, and the ductus arteriosus closes by 96 hours.

Further reading

Murphy PJ. The fetal circulation. *Contin Educ Anaesth Crit Care Pain.* 2005; 5(4): 107–112.

48A: False
48B: True
48C: False
48D: True
48E: True
The functions of the liver are legion and include the metabolism of carbohydrates, proteins and fats. It is also involved in the detoxification of drugs and toxins and storage of glycogen, vitamins (D, E, C and A), iron and copper. Vitamins D, E, K

and A are the fat-soluble vitamins. Fatty acids and lipoproteins are synthesized by the liver and it is the major site for cholesterol and prostaglandin production. The liver is involved in glucose homeostasis through gluconeogenesis, glycogen storage and glycogenolysis. The liver synthesizes many important proteins such as albumin, globulins such as lipoproteins, ferritin, caeruloplasmin, haptoglobins and C-reactive protein.

Further reading

Peterson O. *Lecture Notes: Human Physiology*. 5th ed. Oxford: Wiley-Blackwell; 2006.

49A: True
49B: True
49C: False
49D: False
49E: True

The oesophagus passes through the crura of the diaphragm and joins the stomach just below the diaphragmatic hiatus. The lower oesophageal sphincter (LOS) is formed by the intrinsic circular smooth muscle of the distal 2–4 cm of the oesophagus. The LOS is a physiological sphincter and has a resting pressure of 15–25 mmHg above gastric pressure. It relaxes on swallowing to allow passage of food material from the pharynx to the stomach. A number of factors affect the LOS tone.

Factors that increase the LOS tone include:

- Cholinergic stimulation
- Anticholinesterases (e.g. neostigmine)
- D_2 antagonists (e.g. metoclopramide, prochlorperazine, domperidone)
- Cyclizine
- Succinylcholine

Factors that decrease LOS tone include:

- Swallowing
- Oestrogen, progesterone
- Antimuscarinics (e.g. atropine, glycopyrrolate)
- Dopamine
- Opioids
- Thiopental
- Alcohol

Further reading

Jollife DM. Practical gastric physiology. *Contin Educ Anaesth Crit Care Pain*. 2009; 9(6): 173–177.

50A: True
50B: True
50C: True
50D: True
50E: False

Basal metabolic rate (BMR) is defined as the heat production in a subject in a state of mental and physical rest in a comfortable environment 12 hours after a meal. The BMR of a 70 kg man is 100W, or 2000 kcal·day^{-1}. Body size and surface area are important factors affecting the BMR. Females have a lower BMR due to their higher proportion of body fat. When lean body mass is used as the index of comparison the BMR between sexes is the same. Age is also a factor influencing BMR. It is high in newborns and decreases throughout adult life, typically by about 2% per decade. Eating a meal transiently raises BMR for 4–6 hours by 10–15%. Starvation leads to a decrease in BMR as does living in a hot climate. Other factors increasing BMR include adrenaline and thyroxine. BMR is typically raised about 20% above baseline during pregnancy, particularly in the second and third trimester.

Further reading

Power I, Kam P. *Principles of Physiology for the Anaesthetist*. 2nd ed. London: Hodder Arnold; 2008.

51A: False
51B: True
51C: False
51D: True
51E: False

The mediastinum is the cavity in the thorax that extends superiorly from the thoracic inlet to the diaphragm inferiorly. It is bound anteriorly by the sternum and extends to the vertebral column posteriorly.

The mediastinum is divided into superior and inferior portions. The dividing line is a plane from the sternal angle (angle of Louis) to the body of the fourth thoracic vertebra.

Contents of the superior mediastinum include:

- Veins
  - Brachiocephalic
  - Superior vena cava
- Arteries
  - Brachiocephalic
  - Left common carotid
  - Left subclavian
  - Aortic arch
- Nerves
  - Phrenic and vagus
  - Left recurrent laryngeal
  - Cardiac nerves
  - Sympathetic trunk
- Other
  - Trachea
  - Lymph nodes
  - Oesophagus
  - Thoracic duct
  - Thymic remains

The anterior mediastinum, between the sternum and pericardium, contains sternopericardial ligaments, lymph nodes and thymic remains. The middle mediastinum contains the pericardium, heart, roots of the great blood vessels, trachea, phrenic nerves and lymph nodes.

The posterior mediastinum, between the pericardium and vertebral column, contains the descending aorta, oesophagus, thoracic duct, azygos and hemiazygos veins, vagus nerves, splanchnic nerves, sympathetic trunks and lymph nodes.

The parietal pleura lines the thoracic cage, the diaphragm and the lateral mediastinum. It is sensitive to pain, temperature, touch and pressure. The visceral pleura covers the surface of the lungs and extends into the lung fissures. It is continuous with the parietal pleura at the lung hila. In contrast the visceral pleura is only sensitive to stretch.

Further reading

Snell RS. *Clinical Anatomy*. 7th ed. Philadelphia: Lippincott Williams & Wilkins; 2003.

52A: False
52B: True
52C: True
52D: True
52E: False
The boundaries of the femoral triangle are:

- Superior: inguinal ligament
- Medial: sartorius muscle
- Lateral: abductor longus muscle

The base is the inguinal ligament and its apex is where the sartorius muscle overlies the abductor longus muscle. The floor of the triangle is formed by the pectineus medially and the iliopsoas laterally. The roof is formed by the fascia lata.

The contents from lateral to medial are: the femoral nerve, femoral sheath containing the femoral artery, femoral vein, femoral canal, containing lymph nodes and some lymphatic vessels.

Further reading

Snell RS. *Clinical Anatomy*. 7th ed. Philadelphia: Lippincott Williams & Wilkins; 2003.

53A: False
53B: True
53C: True
53D: True
53E: False
In departmental chest radiographs the patient will usually stand with the plate at their chest and the X-rays are directed from behind. This is a posterior-anterior (PA) film.

Patients in bed will usually have the plate placed behind the back and so will have an anterior-posterior (AP) film. As the plate is closer to the heart in the PA film there will be less magnification of the cardiac outline. In an AP film, the heart can appear artificially enlarged; the widest part of the cardiac outline should be less than half of the width of the thoracic cage. The aortic shadow should be less than 4 cm wide.

When the chest radiograph is taken, the patient will be asked to make a full inspiratory effort. In an adequate inspiratory effort, the right hemidiaphragm should lie below the anterior end of the sixth rib. The right hilum lies at the same level as the horizontal fissure. The left hilum usually lies 1 cm higher than the right hilum.

Further reading

Corne J. *Chest X-Ray Made Easy*. Edinburgh: Churchill Livingstone; 2009.

54A: False
54B: False
54C: False
54D: True
54E: True

The anterior abdominal wall is bordered superiorly by the costal margins, inferiorly by the inguinal ligament and the pubis, and laterally by the mid-axillary line. Regional anaesthesia to block the nerve supply of the anterior abdominal wall is a useful adjunct to analgesia for a variety of procedures involving incision of the anterior abdominal wall.

Three muscles make up the layers of the anterior abdominal wall; each surrounded by a fascial sheath. The most superficial, and largest, is the external oblique; followed by the internal oblique and the transversus abdominis. In the midline lie the two longitudinal rectus muscles.

The abdominal wall is innervated by the anterior rami of T7–L1. The intercostal nerves travel in a plane between the internal oblique and the transversus abdominis muscles, giving off anterior branches to supply the skin (T10 = skin over umbilicus).

The iliohypogastric nerve pierces the internal oblique in front of the anterior superior iliac spine, runs deep to the external oblique and ends supplying the suprapubic skin as well as a gluteal region lateral to the ischial tuberosity. The ilioinguinal nerve traverses the inguinal canal anterior to the spermatic cord. It emerges through the external ring supplying the skin of the scrotum and an area on the upper medial thigh.

Further reading

Ellis H, Feldman S, Harrop-Griffiths W. *Anatomy for Anaesthetists*. 8th ed. Oxford: Wiley-Blackwell; 2003.

Yarwood J, Berrill A. Nerve blocks of the anterior abdominal wall. *Contin Educ Anaesth Crit Care Pain*. 2010; 10(6): 182–186.

55A: False
55B: False
55C: True
55D: False
55E: False
The arterial supply of the spinal cord arises from the anterior and posterior spinal arteries and the radicular branches.

The anterior spinal artery arises from the union of two branches of the vertebral arteries at the level of the foramen magnum, where it descends in the anterior median sulcus. The anterior spinal artery supplies the anterior two-thirds of the spinal cord.

The posterior spinal arteries arise from the posterior inferior cerebellar arteries (PICAs), then each divide into two branches and descend in the lateral aspect of the cord, anterior and posterior to the dorsal nerve roots. The posterior spinal arteries supply the posterior one-third of the cord.

Radicular branches arise segmentally from local arteries, for example, the cervical, intercostal and lumbar arteries, to supply local areas. The great anterior radicular artery of Adamkiewicz supplies the lower two-thirds of the cord.

Further reading

Smith T, Pinnock C, Lin T. *Fundamentals of Anaesthesia*. 3rd ed. Cambridge: Cambridge University Press; 2009. p. 253–258.

56A: False
56B: False
56C: True
56D: False
56E: True
Glycolysis is a 10-reaction series that occurs in the cell cytoplasm. The overall reaction is conversion of one glucose molecule (containing six carbon atoms) to two pyruvate molecules (three carbon atoms each). A net gain of two adenosine triphosphate (ATP) molecules occurs (two ATP are used, four ATP are generated). NADH is produced, which acts as a reducing power in the electron transport chain in the process of oxidative phosphorylation. No oxygen is utilized and no carbon dioxide is produced.

In aerobic conditions, the pyruvate produced is converted to acetyl-CoA, which enters the Krebs (citric acid) cycle. In anaerobic conditions, the pyruvate is converted to lactate, which is converted back to glucose in the liver by the Cori cycle.

Further reading

Power I, Kam P. *Principles of Physiology for the Anaesthetist*. 2nd ed. London: Hodder Arnold; 2008.

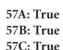

57A: True
57B: True
57C: True
57D: False
57E: True

The autonomic nervous system (ANS) is a collection of nerves and ganglia that are responsible for the maintenance of homeostasis and coordination of the stress response. The ANS controls visceral organs, smooth muscle and secretory glands and is involuntary, hence 'autonomic'.

Sympathetic neurones are thoracolumbar in origin, arising from the lateral horn of the spinal cord grey matter from T1 to L2 segments. Preganglionic fibres leave the cord by the ventral roots, then leave the spinal nerves as white rami communicantes (myelinated B fibres), where they synapse in the sympathetic chain of ganglia. Postganglionic C fibres leave the chain as grey rami communicantes (unmyelinated C fibres) and continue with spinal or visceral nerves to innervate the organ.

Effects of sympathetic stimulation are:

- Ophthalmic: mydriasis, eyelid retraction
- Thoracic: increased heart rate and force of cardiac contraction, pulmonary vasoconstriction, bronchodilation
- Abdominal: increased sphincter tone, reduced peristalsis, redistribution of splanchnic volume due to vasoconstriction
- Pelvic: relaxation of the bladder and sacrum, closing of sphincters, prostate contraction
- Cutaneous: piloerection, vasoconstriction, sweating
- Limbs: skin arteriolar vasoconstriction, skeletal muscle arteriolar vasodilation

Further reading

Menon R. Sympathetic blocks. *Contin Educ Anaesth Crit Care Pain.* 2010; 10(3): 88–92.

58A: True
58B: False
58C: False
58D: False
58E: False

There are 25×10^9 capillaries in the body. Each vessel is on average 1 mm in length, with a diameter of 5–10 micrometres. At rest only 25% of capillaries are open, which leaves a large body of capillaries to be recruited to increase blood flow to an organ by opening pre-capillary sphincters.

The function of capillaries is fluid distribution, and delivery and removal of nutrients and waste.

The movement of fluid across the capillary wall is driven by individual Starling forces; these are hydrostatic and oncotic pressures.

Capillary hydrostatic pressure is the pressure exerted by the fluid within the capillary on the capillary wall. At the arteriolar end, this is 32–36 mmHg and reduces to 12–25 mmHg at the venular end of the capillary. The interstitial hydrostatic pressure is the pressure exerted by the fluid in the interstitium, which is minimal (0 mmHg) or even slightly sub-atmospheric.

The capillary oncotic pressure is the osmotic pressure exerted by large plasma proteins within the capillary and acts to draw fluid into the vessel. This is normally approximately 21–29 mmHg. As the capillary wall is impermeable to plasma proteins and any that may leak out are carried away by lymphatics, the interstitial oncotic pressure is negligible (0 mmHg).

Hence it can be seen that, at the arteriolar end of the capillary, the net filtration pressure promotes fluid passing out of the capillary, whereas, at the venular end, fluid passes into the capillary. This is primarily due to the drop in capillary hydrostatic pressure from the arteriolar to the venular end.

Further reading

Counsell DJ, Rassam SS. Perioperative fluid therapy. *Contin Educ Anaesth Crit Care Pain.* 2005; 5(5): 161–165.

Levick JR, Michel CC. Microvascular fluid exchange and the revised Starling principle. *Cardiovascular Research.* 2010; 87: 198–210.

59A: False
59B: True
59C: False
59D: False
59E: False

Cortisol is a glucocorticoid hormone that is synthesized from 11-deoxycortisol in the zona fasiculata of the adrenal cortex. Cortisol is a steroid hormone that acts on an intracellular nuclear receptor to alter gene transcription and cellular protein synthesis. The production of cortisol is regulated by the pituitary hormone adrenocorticotrophic hormone (ACTH). ACTH acts on the adrenal cortex to increase the conversion of cholesterol to progesterone, thus increasing the production of glucocorticoid hormones. ACTH release is inhibited by cortisol (negative feedback mechanism) and stimulated by corticotrophin releasing hormone (CRH).

There are many effects of cortisol on the body:

- Metabolic
  - Increased hepatic glycogenolysis and gluconeogenesis, fat and protein breakdown, reduced glucose uptake by muscle
- Anti-inflammatory
  - Reduced prostaglandin and leukotriene production, reduced cyclo-oxygenase expression, reduced cytokine, chemokine and tissue plasminogen activator release
- Immunosuppression
  - Reduced cell mediated immunity, T cell production, humoral immunity, antibody production and macrophage release, reduced TNF and interleukin levels
- Foetal development
  - Production of pulmonary surfactant and lung maturity

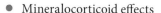

- Mineralocorticoid effects
  - At high levels: sodium and water retention, hypertension, hypokalaemia, metabolic alkalosis
- Haematological
  - Increased red cell and platelet counts
  - Reduced white cell count
- Others
  - Reduced conversion of T_4 to T_3 hormone
  - Osteoporosis
  - Increased cardiovascular sensitivity to circulating catecholamines
  - Impaired production of gastric mucosa

Further reading

Davies M, Hardman J. Anaesthesia and adrenocortical disease. *Contin Educ Anaesth Crit Care Pain.* 2005; 5(4): 122–126.

Power I, Kam P. *Principles of Physiology for the Anaesthetist.* 2nd ed. London: Hodder Arnold; 2008.

60A: False
60B: True
60C: True
60D: False
60E: False
Nitric oxide is synthesized from L-arginine by a group of enzymes called nitric oxide synthases. There are three main subtypes of nitric oxide synthase enzymes, which correspond to the three main functions of endogenous nitric oxide. These are endothelial, neuronal and inducible nitric oxide synthase.

Endothelial nitric oxide is produced by nitric oxide synthase in response to shear stress on the vessel wall. Nitric oxide diffuses into the vascular smooth muscle and activates membrane-bound guanylate cyclase, which catalyzes the formation of cGMP from guanosine triphosphate. cGMP activates protein kinases, causing a reduction in intracellular calcium level and leading to smooth muscle relaxation. The result is reflex local vasodilation in response to mechanical stretch or shear stress on the vessel wall.

Neuronal nitric oxide synthase produces nitric oxide, which acts as a neurotransmitter in non-adrenergic non-cholinergic neurones, which are believed to play a role in matching cerebral blood flow to neural activity and memory. Inducible nitric oxide is produced as part of the inflammatory response, where it has antimicrobial, chemotactic and vasodilator properties. Animal studies suggest inducible nitric oxide plays a role in cellular dysoxia in sepsis and in septic shock.

Further reading

Young D. Nitric oxide. *Contin Educ Anaesth Crit Care Pain.* 2002; 2(6): 161–164.